Praise for *Healthy Kids in an Unhealthy World*

"Dr. Ana Temple is an incredible resource for parents like me. Her new book Healthy Kids in an Unhealthy World has all the tricks you need to survive this over processed world and keep your children healthy and strong."

Vani Hari, AKA The Food Babe, North Carolina

"I have 2 children (10 & 5) and I honestly felt like didn't need this book just because I've read so many other books and thought this would just be the same, but because I follow Dr Temple in IG and love her personality and content, I wanted to support her by purchasing the book. I ended up reading the whole thing in one day, that's how good it is. It's PRACTICAL with very straight forward facts and helpful tips. You're also able to feel so much of her personality through the book, which I love because she is FUNNY! It was a really good refresher for me to read this and motivated me to help my family even more by implementing different tips."

Andy, USA

"I've been following Dr. Ana Maria Temple for years on Instagram and she puts out so much useful information I just had to get her book when it came out. My kids are grown adults and I still find this book completely useful for myself and my husband. It's for everyone, not just parents! I love how it's easy to understand, and she really conveys WHY making healthier choices is important. Everything is backed up with research. Her writing style is funny and authentic which keeps you engaged. Dr. Temple seems aware that one can get stressed trying to make all these changes and encourages you to make small slow adaptations by giving practical solutions. I however, went all in with her suggestions, including ditching added sugar, tossing all my plastic, and trading Teflon for alternatives! She is very persuasive! My biggest shock was about brown rice...I had no idea! With its charts it makes it a great guide to keep on hand for future reference. I find it could be improved with wider margins for notes and an index for quick referencing."

Gwenn, USA

D1662310

"Amazing book packed full of actionable tips for raising a family in today's world. As a mom, who is busy working, I appreciated Dr Temple's honesty that keeping her family healthy and happy took effort and hard work. I have shared this book with friends already! Super helpful! Thanks for writing this, Dr Temple!"

Sylvia, USA

"It can feel so hard to do the right things to keep your kids healthy. Limiting video games, feeding them vegetables instead of fast food and water instead of soda - it isn't always easy! Dr Temple has a wealth of PRACTICAL tips that really work, learned through experience from working with her patients and from raising her own kids. Her advice is sprinkled with lots of humor (spoiler alert: her family isn't perfect!) to help us be inspired to do our best as parents (even when we're not perfect either....)"

Deb, USA

"Such an easy read that gets right to the necessary info, in a way that is still light-hearted, funny, and relatable! It was incredibly encouraging to see that Dr. Temple's family had to make changes gradually, over time, in order to have a healthy lifestyle that was *sustainable*. It is so encouraging when real people have real solutions, that really do make a difference if you choose to stick with it. So thankful I stumbled across Dr. Temple, and purchased this book! Chapters are also laid out in bite sized, easily digestible, sections. Highly recommend to anyone wanting to make practical, healthy changes, and apply them in a maintainable way."

Monica, USA

"This book is a must read for everyone kids or no kids! I have really enjoyed learning! She has a great sense of humor, very authentic and real and extremely informative and helpful. I feel so encouraged with my family's health journey and I am more aware and knowledgeable on how to continue in the direction to choosing a healthy lifestyle for us and teaching it to my children!"

Andrew, USA

"Such a great book, full of easy and practical advices for implementing gradually small changes at home and improve our family health and immune system to be at its best if needed. It's a great summary of important health topics in Coronavirus times, explained in an easy and funny way (and not feeling guilty of not being perfect parents). What I love most are the practical tips that are easy to implement at home. Would definitely recommend to anyone interested in improving its health and immune system."

April, USA

"I loved this book! I love her layout (lots of bullet points for easy quick reading for a busy mom like me!). Very easy to understand and gave me SO MANY easy tips for adapting our family into a more healthy lifestyle. We are fairly healthy already, but there is soo much more to it. Dr. Ana-Maria gives her real life experience (she's made ALL the mistakes we've all made!) and gives us hope that we can be healthier and it's actually possible! Very encouraged by her motherhood journey and excited for any and all other books she writes!! Thank you Dr. Ana-Maria!"

Michelle, USA

"If you want to protect yourself and your family from all the greedy unhealthy chemical inclusions in your food, this lady has all the answers for you. All it takes is constant vigilance and amazing discipline and you can protect yourself and your children from food additives that first do you harm."

Sharon, USA

"I love the bullet points and how easy she makes the information to understand. Often it feels like you need a degree to decode research and books on this, not this one! She presents the facts and then gives solutions. It can be done all at once or little by little. I would highly recommend this for any parents but especially busy ones trying to maximize time and learning."

Aimee, USA

The material in this book is for informational purposes only and is not intended as a substitute for the advice and care of your physician or dentist. As with all new diet and wellness regiments the nutrition and lifestyle programs described in this book should be followed only after first consulting with your physician or dentist to make sure it is appropriate for your individual circumstances. The authors and publisher expressly disclaim responsibility for any adverse effects that may result from the use or application of the information contained in this book.

ISBN 978-1-7356222-2-4

Ebook ISBN 978-1-7356222-3-1

Practical Parenting Tips for
Picky Eating, Toxin Reduction, and
Stronger Immune Systems

Healthy Kids
In An Unhealthy World

DR. ANA-MARIA TEMPLE, MD

CONTENTS

Introduction   11

Temple Family Timeline   16

Current State of Children's Health   21

The Immune System   23

Pillar I - NUTRITION   25

1	A Family That Eats Together	31
2	But I Hate It!!!	37
3	You Can Teach Old Buds New Tricks	49
4	Don't Kale My Vibe	55
5	Snack Shark Attack	59
6	No Pop-Tart Party Here	65
7	Let 'Em Steal Your Lucky Charms	69
8	A Whopper of a Bad Decision	73
9	Don't Shop 'til You Drop	79
10	Old MacDonald Had an Organic Farm	83
11	So Many Fish in the Sea	91
12	Where's the Beef?	99
13	The Chicken or the Egg?	107
14	Need an Oil Change?	113
15	Arsenic for Dummies	121
16	You Lyte Up My Life	127
17	Keeping It Real	133

18   Don't Let Your Sweet Emotion Get the Best of You   139

19   Pour Some Sugar on Me   149

20   Sugar Monsters   153

21   Ho-Ho-Hold It Together During the Holidays   159

22   Leave the Extra Baggage Behind   163

PILLAR II - STRESS   169

23   Banishing the Burnout   173

PILLAR III - SLEEP   181

24   Channel Your Sleeping Beauty   185

PILLAR IV - MOVEMENT   191

25   They've Got to Move It Move It   195

PILLAR V - ENVIRONMENT   201

26   Here Comes the Sun   205

27   Stop Bugging Me   213

28   The Dirty on Keeping Clean   221

29   Fluorination Station   227

30   Life with Plastic, Not Fantastic   233

31   I'll Take Mine Sunny Side Up   239

Acknowledgements   245

References   247

Dedication

I know, I know, this should be a list of names. But I like to make my own rules. This book has been created from the bond and love of a family. How corny is this start? Stay with me.

In December 2016, on a beautiful day in New Zealand I sat sipping coffee with my friend Daina from Sweden. She looked over her cup of coffee at me and said, "I cannot wait for your book." I protested immediately "There is no book. I have zero interest in writing a book, as in a negative 10 desire on a scale from 1-10." She just looked at me, shrugged and said "Okay, but I want the first copy when you do write it." The nerve of some people.

Three years later, it became clear that I needed to write a book and I'd better get on with it. I called several publishing houses, did my research on this topic, became completely overwhelmed, crawled into a corner, curled up in the fetal position, and gave up on the idea.

Some months later, the book thing was still nagging at me. Over the past 19 years I had raised 3 children. I learned a lot from these little humans and their endless needs and along the way I accumulated a lot of parenting material. Furthermore, I had already written many posts and blogs on how to raise healthy kids. It was time to put it all together in a book.

Over dinner one night, my husband, John, and I looked at each other while discussing this book and we both concluded that my sister-in-law, Jen, should edit the book. Of note, I have tried to convince my sister-in-law to become a book editor for 20 years. I guess if she wasn't going to do it organically, we were going to make her. Thus, Jen became my editor-in-chief. As she was pouring over the pages one day, my niece, Mary Kate, an English major, walked in and was horrified at some of my diction and grammar. I guess even after 36 years in this country, I am still struggling with the English language.

Later, my mother-in-law got wind of the project and she put her two cents in as well. At one point, as I read my chapter on cleaning solutions to my dog, he was so inspired by the content he began enthusiastically licking his butt. I took this as a positive sign and kept on writing. However, the book had a dry feel, so John's wittiness was called upon to liven things up. His first contribution was the proposed title: "How I Stole the Joy from My Husband's Life." Needless to say, that did not make the cut. Since he was so hilarious, he was put in charge of several exciting things like charts and formatting.

This book is more than advice on how to raise healthy kids. It is a manuscript interlaced with a family's love and dedication. As a family, we came together, despite previous resentments and miscommunications, for one common purpose, to change children's lives. We are all on a journey of self-discovery, family bonding, and nutritional rebirth. Know that we are with you every step of the way.

Introduction

In Bucharest, Romania, circa 1978, my 3-year-old sister, Roxy, suffered from chronic abdominal pain and failure to thrive. I distinctly remember my mom sitting on the floor with Roxy in her arms, rocking and crying. We went to many doctors and Roxy had to take various disgusting medications. Some of those concoctions were given to me, an innocent bystander, just in case. At one point, they even believed Roxy had worms.

Eventually, she was diagnosed with celiac disease. My mom had to find gluten-free food in communist Romania. Let me explain, we hardly had access to food at all, much less gluten-free food. For example, we would stand in lines for hours to get two sticks of butter, my mom in one line, me in another. My dad would go to the butcher in the morning to get a number and then return later in the day to pick up whatever was available. Fortunately, there was a black market for just about everything behind the iron curtain.

Because Roxy was so picky, my mom would spend hours making the right food with specific consistencies, and then battle with Roxy to eat it. It went on and on. It was during this time, amidst tears, pain, doctor visits, and medications, that I found solace while playing with my baby dolls. I could make them better. They were happy and pain free. Food didn't hurt them anymore. The dolls were at peace because I was their doctor.

At the age of five, my mission took shape: to help kids feel better. I wanted to become a pediatrician. Not just a doctor, but a doctor who helped prevent children from getting sick.

Pursuit of higher of education for my sister and I was one of the many reasons my non-English speaking dad defected to the United States in 1981. By day he cleaned bathrooms at Bloomingdales while he learned English at night school. After three years of ostracization by the communists, my mom, sister, and I were released to America on permanent visas.

My mom always cooked meals from scratch, but she also wanted us to acclimate to the American way of living. Thus, Apple Jacks, Lean Cuisine, Keebler cookies, and the like were in our pantry for the taking. In addition to the stress that comes along with moving to a foreign country, I started sixth grade unable to speak English. Once I started learning the language, I was mortified to let other kids see I was missing two front teeth thanks to a family genetic defect.

I was bullied because I was different and progressively developed anxiety and anorexia nervosa. Food became my enemy. Although doctors diagnosed me as "recovered" from my eating disorder, my diet deteriorated in college from unlimited access to cafeteria goodies and, of course, alcohol. By the time I started medical school, my breakfast consisted of Diet Coke and Pop-Tarts. I usually ate crummy hospital food or my remaining Pop-Tart for lunch, and then a "homemade" dinner. By homemade, I mean frozen pizzas and burritos, TV dinners, and many of the other typical American ready-made meals.

Despite my food craziness, I was always an active person, though not very athletic. I always had a hunch that food was at the core of my issues, but without any guidance during undergraduate school or from my medical school training, I ignored my instincts. I was thin and "healthy." I mean, taking MiraLAX daily for years is normal, right?

Fast forward to 2007. I was working a full-time job as a hospitalist in Charlotte, North Carolina and I had three children; three very sick children. They were 2, 4, and 6 years old.

The 2-year-old had allergies so severe he could not attend Easter egg hunts because if he went outside, his eyes would swell shut, his body would be covered in hives, and he would writhe on the floor in discomfort.

The 6-year-old had asthma acute enough to require daily steroids, eczema requiring daily topical steroids, and seasonal allergies needing daily medications. If she got a cold it would turn into an ear infection, sinusitis, or croup requiring steroids and antibiotics.

The 4-year-old was plagued by ADHD since the day he was born. He was also disgusting. He had the kind of green snot that horrifies parents. People often wondered what kind of mother would let her child walk out of the house in such a state. There were not enough tissues in Costco to take care of those boogers.

One day, I took this three-ring circus to the doctor to discuss alternate strategies for their illnesses. Unfortunately, this was what they said: "For the little one, there are no more drugs to give him. He is already on five medications. The only option is to start allergy shots." He was 2 years old.

"The princess can take daily inhaled steroids to keep her asthma under control, she will need to use daily topical steroids to keep her eczema under control, and if she also takes daily allergy meds to keep her asthma and eczema under control, she should be fine.

"As for the snotty one, we don't know what to do with him. He's just gross." OK maybe I wasn't listening by the time we discussed the third one! I was stunned. I was five years into my medical practice and I had no idea what to do. I walked out of that office and my mom instinct said: "No way will I allow these three young children to be on daily medications for the rest of their lives!"

One week later, I attended a nutrition lecture at one of my children's schools. It was at that time, 7:30 A.M. on a Tuesday morning that the fog lifted and I identified the issue behind my kid's chronic disease. All the nutritionist talked about was sugar.

Realizing that food was hurting my children (a common theme in my life after Roxy), I went home that night and cleaned out the pantry as the kids watched in horror. Out went the Lucky Charms, the Cinnamon Toast Crunch, the Pop-Tarts, mac and cheese, chicken nuggets, juice boxes, chocolate milk, and orange peanut butter crackers. You name it, we were eating it, and into the trash it all went.

It was at this time that I became an outcast. No one liked me! No one, including my husband, John. We fought over food all the time. "Food has nothing to do with chronic disease. I ate this stuff and I am fine" John said. My friends thought I had lost my mind.

My 24 medical practice partners at that time said, "Where is the medical evidence behind these ideas?" I said, "I don't know where the medical evidence is behind this weird stuff, but I know in my mom gut that this is the right thing to do. It cannot be wrong to get rid of this garbage food and eat fruits and vegetables."

Over the next five years, I persevered despite all the criticism and the naysayers. Throughout those years, my kids got better. Slowly they stopped needing antibiotics, then steroids, and eventually chronic meds became unnecessary. Within five years, our family experienced a 180-degree turnaround. Their immune systems were humming along better than ever. In 2016, nine years later, we moved to New Zealand with no health insurance, no doctors, no medication, and no fear of chronic disease. The kids thrived. No one got sick from the new environment. They climbed the highest mountains and bungee jumped off the tallest bridges.

I realized over this 12-year journey that we can turn chronic disease around by building up the immune system and getting rid of toxic medications that suppress our immune systems. Nutrition and lifestyle are at the core of children's wellness.

As my children got better, my medical practice changed. I noticed that what I was doing was helping my kids, thus I started giving my patients different medical advice. They also started asking different questions which led me to more research. Low and behold, I found Functional Medicine.

In New Zealand, I had the opportunity to practice medicine without fear of malpractice and without patient satisfaction scores on Yelp. 90% of my patients got better without medications. Once I arrived back in the U.S., I did not want to practice medicine the same way I had before. So, I opened my own practice where I successfully started treating and preventing chronic disease with nutrition and lifestyle modifications.

Two years into my new clinical practice, a global pandemic hit. My families were prepared. Those with chronic illnesses which would have put them at great risk for adverse outcomes from COVID-19 no longer suffered. Weakened immune systems were strengthened. Parents who were previously riddled with anxiety and worried about their children's well-being were equipped with the tools they needed to protect their families from any viral illness that came their way.

The best treatment for chronic disease and viral illnesses is prevention. Prevention begins with a strong immune system. The immune system is built and reinforced with Five Pillars: Nutrition, Sleep, Movement, Inner Peace, and Environment. We must stop waiting for disease to rear its ugly head before we change our ways. Poor food choices and our lifestyles are hurting our children and many of us are still unaware of these issues. While we are months into the pandemic, many of us are still confused about what we need to do.

I hope this book inspires, educates, and empowers you to better care for your family.

The Temple Family Timeline

As I previously mentioned, our family's health journey began in 2007. But what did it look like? What did we do first? How did I convince my people to go along with the plan rather than revolt? I put together the timeline of our journey to illustrate that change doesn't happen overnight. All journeys begin with a first step.

2007

- **Day One** - Tuesday, March 13, 2007 at 7:30 A.M., I had my "aha" moment and my mindset changed. I threw out all the garbage from my pantry: mac and cheese in a box, Cheetos, Doritos, peanut butter crackers (yep, the gross orange ones), Jell-O, etc. My kids stared in horror at all the food going into the trash. That was day one.

- **Food coloring** - I got rid of food coloring from the pantry. It is harder than you think. An easy rule of thumb: if the box is colorful on the outside, the items inside are almost always artificially colored.

- **Fruits and veggies** - I added a fruit to every lunch and a vegetable or fruit to every dinner.

- **Fast food was abolished** - No more fast-food other than Subway.

2008

- **Juice Plus** - The family started taking Juice Plus.

- **Juice and chocolate milk were discontinued** - Juice and chocolate milk were removed from lunch boxes over a period of a few weeks.

- **Fruit and vegetables became snacks** - Fruits or vegetables became mandatory for anyone hungry for a snack. To earn the opportunity to eat a processed food/snack, one had to eat some form of a plant.

2009

- **The Vitamix** - John bought what he described as "a ridiculously over-priced blender" for me on Mother's Day. (He now worships the blender)

- **More fruits and veggies** - Fruits and vegetables became part of breakfast.

- **Artificial food ingredients were removed** - Food label reading became an art form. If I couldn't read it, we didn't eat it. I chose to eliminate one snack food at a time to save my sanity.

- **Soda was gone** - I gave up soda. My water drinking skyrocketed.

2010

- **More fruits and veggies** - Fruit and vegetable portion sizes increased and became present at breakfast, lunch, after-school snack, and dinner. Veggies became mandatory on all Subway sandwiches. No more chips, only fruit slices at Subway.

- **Organic food** – I began transitioning to organic fruits and veggies and organic milk.

- **Drinks were simplified** - Water and milk became the only drinks in the house, ever.

- **Travel food** - We began packing food for road trips to avoid fast food restaurants and garbage eating on the road.

2011

- **Low fat items were removed** – We transitioned to full-fat organic dairy of any kind.

- **Omega 3s** – We incorporated Omega 3s into our daily diet through fish oil, flax seed, hemp seeds, or chia seeds in smoothies.

- **Meat labels were scrutinized** – We moved to grass-fed meat, nitrite-free bacon, and turkey breast without colors or additives for lunches, thanks to *Food Inc*, the movie.

- **Organic eggs** - These became the norm.

- **Vacation eating was adjusted** - On vacation we started eating like our everyday meals. No more kids' meals or menus.

2012

- **Gluten free** - I gave up gluten. People! That may have been the hardest thing in the world because I love the taste of beer, but my bloating was out of control.

- **Marriage counseling** - This is a very important step in a healthy lifestyle. We were struggling and on the brink of divorce.

- **A holistic chef was engaged for meals on nights when we both worked** – Part of our marital rehab plan included help with dinner. I hired Chef Sherri with The Seasonal Kitchen. I know, it sounds "bougie," but thanks to Sherri, I learned how to prep meals, our vegetable repertoire increased by 100%, and we started eating fish regularly. My stress level decreased, meal prep became enjoyable, and my food shopping got even cleaner.

2013

- **VSL 3** - I was introduced to VSL3, a probiotic. Within 48 hours, I developed normal bowel habits for the first time in 22 years without medications. I was stunned!

2014

- **Chemicals** – We transitioned to chemical free cleaners.

- **Soap** – We cut out antibacterial soap.

2015

- **Skin care** – We began choosing cleaner products.

- **Think Dirty** - I started using the Think Dirty app to evaluate my skin care and cosmetics.

2016

- **Stress Reduction** - John quit his job and we moved to New Zealand, where serenity reigns and work-life balance is an actual reality.

2017

- **John's sleep** – Significant improvement with less stress. Thanks, New Zealand living!

- **My sleep** - I finally weaned myself of Clonazepam (Xanax). It helped me to stay asleep during our rough marriage days. Despite great sleep hygiene habits, many regular medications trials, and acupuncture, I struggled to wean off. With the help of functional medicine, that mission was accomplished.

2018

- **Back in the U.S.** - We arrived back in the U.S. to our giant home filled with stuff. *A lot* of stuff. After four months of attempting to live in the footprints of our previous life, we decided to sell our house and give away 75% of our stuff to our family and friends. Catharsis!

- **Down-sizing** - We moved into a 3-bedroom apartment.

- **New beginnings** - I started my clinic, Integrative Health Carolinas. I began my mission to change the face of healthcare by preventing disease and treating chronic disease with nutrition and lifestyle modifications. John went back to his previous practice with a new attitude and new goals.

- **Marriage counselor** – Counselor #3 helped us overcome many leftover resentments and deep unresolved feelings that were poisoning our relationship. The treatment plan: no alcohol for 6 weeks which happened to be during Thanksgiving and Christmas.

2019

- **Fresh start** - John realized that a traditional orthopedic practice was not for him. He quit in December 2019 and found a new path, a new beginning.
- **TV** - I took my mission to the television stage. I started traveling across the country to bring awareness to children's wellness.

2020

- **Pandemic** - A pandemic took hold of the world.
- **Slowing down** - Thanks to the pandemic, our family slowed down. I realized that, once again, I had allowed myself to get swept up into a crazy pace of life. If we are going to be honest, I had jumped in with both feet!
- **A gift** - My college daughter had to come home and I got to have all my kids under one roof for three extra months.
- **The team** - John and I joined forces and launched two online courses: The Eczema Transformation and Virtual Pediatrician.
- **Many have cursed this difficult year. I chose to use 2020 as my inspiration for great change.**

2021

- **Zoom School** – we watched our middle schooler struggle with zoom school and become a complete couch potato with no desire to socialize or separate from YouTube
- **New beginnings** – we moved into our new house, a smaller and less cluttered creation, with greener building products, and we got a reverse osmosis filter

- **New School Year Started** – and we continued to talk about the same thing as in 2020. Masks, vaccines, Plexiglas, hand sanitizers. Still no mention of vegetables or sunshine. Is anyone paying attention?

The Current State of Children's Health

Before we delve into the immune system and tips for raising healthy kids, we need to understand that we have a huge problem: chronic disease in children. Most people have been petrified by the 2020 pandemic caused by a virus called COVID-19, but very few are aware of the pandemic that has been ravaging our children for decades: chronic disease.

At this point, you may look at your little darling playing happily with Legos or looking at the iPad and think, how is this book going to help me? My kid is fine. We are fine.

We are not fine. Our kids are sick and getting sicker.

- 1 in 8 children dealt with chronic disease in 1994. [1]
- 1 in 3 children struggled with chronic disease in 2015. [2]
- Let me simplify. The rates more than doubled in just over 20 years.

This means, if you have 3 children, one of your children has or will soon have, a chronic issue. We can wait for that to happen, or we can start by making some changes.

Let's break it down a bit more. According to the CDC:

- 1 in 5 kids have eczema (rates in 1970 were 1 in 15). [3]
- 1 in 10 kids are estimated to have ADHD. [4]
- 1 in 59 kids are diagnosed with an autism spectrum disorder (rates in 2010 were 1 in 88). [5]
- 1 in 5 school-aged kids are overweight. [6]
- 1 in 6 U.S. children ages 2 through 8 have a diagnosed mental,

behavioral, or developmental disorder. [7]

- 1 in 13 kids have food allergies. [8]
- 1 in 13 kids under the age of 18 have asthma. [9]
- 1 in 6 kids have type 2 diabetes. The rates of type 2 diabetes were near zero in 1990. [10]

I hear you. This is scary and you're worried that this book is going to complicate your already busy life. There are so many decisions, products, foods, ideas, cosmetics, and parenting suggestions to consider. It all culminates in decision fatigue. The consequence of decision fatigue is to do nothing and maintain the status quo. Instead, let me help.

The main purpose of this book is to simplify your life. I will give you information about why I propose the changes I do and how you can implement them. Within each chapter you will find a simple takeaway that you can implement today. If you are in a rush and just need the vital takeaways, navigate to the end of the chapter where you will find my **Rule of 5**. These are main points to take from each chapter and apply to your life for healthier families.

The Immune System

Your Secret Weapon Against Chronic Disease and Viral Illnesses

Once upon a time, in the year 2020, there was a pandemic that took over the world. The culprit: a virus named **COVID-19**. The experts tried to decipher the inaccurate numbers. Fights over to mask or not to mask broke out. People were trapped in their houses in the name of quarantine. Arguments ensued over plexiglass dividers, social isolation, and who started the pandemic. And on and on it went. Mass confusion reigned. So many questions were posed and it seemed like there were very few answers. Until this book.

The situation is actually very simple. COVID-19, like the flu, is just a virus. The human body has defended itself against viruses since the dawn of time with... drumroll please: the immune system. If the immune system is strong, the human body wins. If the virus is stronger, the human body suffers. Unfortunately, as usual, the humans who think they know more than Mother Nature have confused the general public with a lot of noise and incorrect information. It's time we go back to the basics and understand how **The 5 Pillars** are the solution to preventing chronic disease and defending us against viruses:

1. Nutrition

2. Stress

3. Sleep

4. Movement

5. Environment

The power lies within each of us as humans to build a strong immune system. It is our responsibility to make this a priority!

Pillar I

NUTRITION

Nutrition and The Immune System

Food is a basic human need. When hunger strikes, we eat food and simply move on. Does it really matter what we eat? How do our food choices contribute to chronic disease or illnesses? I'm sure you have heard that eating fruits and vegetables will keep you "healthy" but what does that even mean?

Our health in large part depends on our body's ability to manufacture quality cells, hormones, enzymes, etc. The building blocks of that manufacturing process are the macronutrients, micronutrients, vitamins, minerals, and antioxidants found in food. [6] If the supply chain provides the body with poor materials (garbage food), it will make an inferior product (garbage cells).

The immune system, for example, is very complex. To simplify, it is made up of two branches and many types of cells and proteins whose purpose is to keep foreign invaders such as colds, flu or COVID19 at bay. Neutrophils, lymphocytes, eosinophils and basophils are examples of immune system cells. All cells grow, repair themselves, and die. Here are some examples:

- Neutrophils take about 1 week to regenerate. [1]
- Lymphocytes last 1 week to months; some are long-lived and last years. [2]
- Basophils renew themselves in 60-70 hours. [3]
- Eosinophils live 18 hours to 6 days. [4]
- You get the picture.
- What do all cells use to rebuild, repair, and grow?

-- Insert Jeopardy music here --

Cells need more than energy in the form of calories, they need building materials such as zinc, vitamin D, and vitamin C. Each cell has specific channels and receptors that depend on the aforementioned vitamins and minerals. However, cells do not have receptors for monosodium glutamate, polysorbate 80, blue 1, etc. Calling on all people who ever took a biology course: Where in the cell cycle did you learn that dimethylpolysiloxane is used? Have you ever heard of this word? It's an antifoaming agent in French fries in a beloved fast food. My point is this: your cells cannot be expected to decipher a lab-made chemical designed to prevent foam in food. Man-made chemicals have the capacity to injure our cells, create chaos, interfere with cell to cell messaging, and damage hormones. This leads to a polluted system of sick and confused cells with inappropriate signaling. Sick cells trigger inflammation in the lungs (asthma), mistakenly allow bad cells to grow (cancer), and render immune cells ineffective (COVID-19 sickness).

The body is under attack daily. It needs to work quickly, efficiently, and effectively to protect and defend itself against invaders like viruses, bacteria, fungus, and cancer. Every time we sit down for a meal or a snack, we make the choice to either enhance or tarnish this amazing machine, the human body.

Food intake is perhaps the most difficult habit to change. It is the human need most tainted by chemicals, marketing, and money from the food industry. Food is not simply nutrition; it has social implications, deeply ingrained cultural habits, and immensely polarizing biases. For example, people *love* their cereal. People identify themselves by their favorite cereal. No one identifies themselves by their favorite vegetable (unless you are my patient).

Here is what the medical literature has to say on this topic:

- Foods high in protein (macronutrient), vitamin C, vitamin D, vitamin E, and fiber can reduce inflammation associated with viral illnesses such as COVID-19. People eating diets low in micronutrients such as vitamin A and zinc have higher risk of infection. [5]

- People who ate a diet full of fruits and vegetables were less likely to catch COVID and less likely to be hospitalized from the virus, according to a recent paper published by Harvard Medical School. [5a]

- Large doses of sugar, more than 100 grams, weaken the immune system 1 to 2 hours after consumption. The effects can last for up to 5 hours, likely contributing to the onslaught of colds seen after a kiddie birthday party. [6] 100grams of sugar is found in 10 ounces of orange juice, 1 can of soda, or 2 slices of sheet cake.

- Healthy young men who ate 50 grams of sugar from glucose and carbohydrates like white bread and pasta, had a significant increase in inflammatory markers responsible for chronic disease. [7] 50 grams are in 1 cup of cooked pasta, 2 slices of white bread, or 28 jellybeans.

- Children who started eating a Mediterranean diet used 87% fewer antibiotics and had 56.7% fewer colds when compared to the time before they changed their diets. [8]

- Children with recurrent ear infections underwent food elimination based on testing. 70% of kids had resolution of ear infections. Food reintroduction in the same children caused recurrence of ear infections in 66% of the children. [9,10]

- Sudanese children with the highest intake of Vitamin A from green leafy and non-leafy vegetables had 25-45% lower risk of experiencing diarrhea, cough with fever, or measles [11]

1

A Family That Eats Together...

Making Family Dinners a Priority

We have always tried to make sitting down for dinner as a family a top priority. As our family transitioned away from processed foods to healthier options, I felt inspired to experiment with new recipes and tastes. Unfortunately, my foray into new cooking techniques occasionally spawned some dinners even my dog would reject. But I expected the family to sit and "enjoy" the meal without comment, regardless of the dish. Compounding my cooking woes was the fact that my husband literally ate every meal with a huge box of Cheez-Its under his chair, attempting to sneak crackers between bites of my creations. The children quickly caught on to his scheme and would desperately plead for "cracks" like prisoners being fed gruel. Oh, how far we have come!

Sharing meals as a family is crucial for proper child development. Let's look at the various stages and discuss why breaking bread together is vital to raising healthy kids.

TODDLERS

- **Toddlers and small children are learning new vocabulary.** The recommended number of words per day spoken to and in front of a toddler/preschooler is 3000 or more. Dinner time can introduce kids to 1000 or more simple and complex words. This is more than the exposure received from books being read aloud. Words heard on TV or other electronics do not count toward the total daily requirements. [1]

- **Healthier food is consumed when eaten at the family table.** Young children are exposed to more fruits, vegetables, and healthy proteins at the family dinner table. Parents are less likely to present foods such as soda, crackers, fried foods, and snacks at this time. Children are less likely to become picky eaters when presented with family dinners.

- **Teenage habits are formed during toddler years.** Manners and skills such as taking turns speaking at the table are critical life lessons.

SCHOOL-AGED CHILDREN

- **Eating together as a family has multiple health and social benefits.**[1] More family mealtimes result in higher academic achievements in school. Children who have regular family meals also tend to experience fewer issues with anxiety and asthma. In addition, eating family dinners with the TV off has been associated with healthier weights in children in the short and long terms in multiple countries. And setting and clearing the table allows young children to contribute to household chores.

TEENS

- **Family meals increase the psychological well-being of teens thereby decreasing depression, suicidal ideation, and anxiety and improving overall mood and outlook.** [1,2] Family mealtimes result in a 75% reduction in risky teen behaviors such as smoking marijuana, drinking alcohol, sex, teen pregnancy, smoking tobacco, dropping out of school, violence, and eating disorders. Teens who are victims of cyberbullying also adjust better and overcome these issues more quickly and successfully when they are part of regular family meals. Family dinners result in teens getting better grades in school. [1]

- **Children learn respect.** Being respectful, sitting quietly, listening while others speak, and contributing to a conversation without autocorrect, emojis, and selfies are vital life lessons for adult interactions and career success.

- **Teens who eat regularly with their parents grow up to eat healthier diets as adults.** [1,3] Teens are often drawn to junk foods, soda, and fast foods. Family meals provide them with more fruits, veggies, vitamins and nutrients.

Steps to Creating a Family Dinner

Choose Optimal Days

Start with days when family members have the fewest activities. Set those family mealtimes in stone and make no exceptions. The goal is a minimum of 5 family meals per week. Remember, few activities run late on Saturday and Sunday nights. Use these nights for family time.

- **If you come home late from work every evening, pick a night to reverse the routine.** Give kids a healthy snack in the early afternoon (fruits, veggie, protein, not crackers), do homework, take baths, read books, and complete other nighttime routines and then eat dinner. There is no rule about what comes first. In our house, during busy sports seasons, we ate at 8:30 some nights. We just made it work.

Finish Work at Work

Parents often work late, way too late to allow kids to wait up for them. For instance, my husband and I are both physicians and we have tons of charts to complete, phone calls to make, letters to write, administrative emails to read, blah blah blah. However, we have a set time when we must be home for family. It works 90% of the time. This means:

- Some emails must wait.

- We must occasionally leave meetings early.

- Charts are left for the next day.

- Blogs are postponed to another time.

- There are always critical deadlines, important meetings, and important projects at work. Prioritize some nights differently.

> **ProTip**
> *The most important project you will ever create is a well-adjusted, productive member of society, your child. The most important meeting, that should never be cancelled - Family Dinner.*

Manage Electronics

- No television. No tablets or cell phones on or under the table. Catch up on the daily news, sports scores and television programs another time. Now is the time to pay attention to the kids. The greatest and latest news affecting your life is happening every day around your table. The most critical score is on the latest school project, test, or current report card.

Talk to Your Kids

- Conversation is an important part of dinner time. Make a great effort to keep lines of communication positive and interactive. It may be difficult at first, but like anything else, practice makes perfect. What to talk about?

Our favorite Dinner Ice Breaker: Rose, Bud, Thorn:

- Rose: Share the best part of your day.
- Bud: Share something you are looking forward to.
- Thorn: Share an unpleasant part of your day.

Other Dinner Discussion Ideas:

- Who did you help today?
- Who did you play with?
- What was your biggest struggle today?

- Challenge each person around the table to do something the next day such as: open the door for someone, talk to a person with whom you rarely interact, play with a child who gets left out.

Traveling Parents

In some families, a parent travels or can rarely be home on time, despite good intentions. In this case, I urge the parent at home to sit down with the kids whether they are eating or not. Sitting down for fifteen minutes with the kids, rather than doing other things while the children eat can create a solid connection. That kind of connection can be difficult to accomplish during carpool, story time, or other points during the day.

Aim for family dinners at least 5 nights per week.

For my mega list of shopping items from Costco, Walmart, Trader Joe's, Target, Aldi, etc. scan the code for my book resources page.

2
But I Hate It!!!
Picky Eaters and How to Feed Them

In 20 years of practicing medicine, I have never seen nor heard of a child starving to death with a plate of food sitting in front of them. Yet, I continued to panic when my picky eater child refused dinner because it wasn't one of the three food products he would eat. I was convinced he would lie in bed that night writhing with hunger pains and crying out until social services showed up and hauled me away to poor-parenting prison. My husband convinced me it was time for some tough love. You can imagine my delight when, after several nights in a row of going to bed hungry, he magically began to eat some of whatever we served. Remember, you are not running a restaurant for these small people who live in your home.

I've addressed the importance of family dinners. There are many challenges to this special ritual, but none are more frustrating than picky eaters. It's an issue most parents will face at some point. Let's start from the beginning and move through the teens. My research and personal experience indicate that habits formed in the early years continue into the teen years. One of my favorite sayings is, "Do not start and/or endorse habits that you don't plan on following through in the long run." Excellent parenting advice, simple and true, but it can be tough to follow in the midst of crying and whining children.

BABIES SIX MONTHS AND OLDER

At This Point, Solid Food Introduction Is On Its Way.

- **I recommend fruits and veggies as the first foods for babies.** When training taste buds, never start with processed flakes in a box. The food industry has added iron to this useless creation, to make us believe that we are feeding our children food. Go for the good stuff: fruits and veggies. Of note, green leafy veggies are a natural source of iron. By six months, I encourage parents to offer babies all foods except cow's milk, sugar, and raw honey. Fruits, veggies, eggs, fish, meat, peanut butter, cheese, yogurt, etc. may all be introduced.

- **Highchairs should be used regularly.** Around this stage in the feeding journey, I suggest babies sit in a highchair with the parents at the dinner table.

- **By 9 months, babies should be sampling the parental meals.** Whatever meal the parents have prepared for themselves can be put into a blender or food processor and pureed for little gums: eggs, sausage, spinach or chicken, rice, and broccoli, dinner, lunch, or break-fast, it can all be pureed. This way, babies taste the salt and spices at the family table and begin the transition to real food. Ok to play around with chunkier foods if your child can chew and more teeth emerge.

- **Beware of sugar laden baby foods.** Under the age of 2yrs old I recommend ZERO added sugar in babies' diets. Finger foods marketed for babies are often laden with ingredients such as: sugar and fruit juice. Even if organic these ingredients train our babies' taste buds for carbs and sugar, which leads to picky toddlers.

TODDLERS

Growth During Toddler Years Slows Down and So Do Their Appetites.

- In the first year of life kids double or even triple their birth weight. They are hungry for foods and ready to try anything. They turn 15 months old and begin to chuck food on the floor, refusing to eat anything that is not white (bread, bananas, apple sauce, toast, and pasta). Frustration rises throughout the home.

Let's look at a growth chart and understand the biology of food refusal:

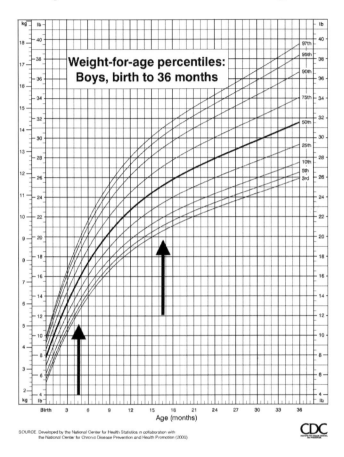

**Weight-for-age percentiles:
Boys, birth to 36 months**

SOURCE: Developed by the National Center for Health Statistics in collaboration with
the National Center for Chronic Disease Prevention and Health Promotion (2000)

CDC

Look at the weight line between 15 and 18 months (toddler) and compare it to the line between 3 and 6 months (baby). Notice how flat the toddler line is compared to the baby line. Looking at this chart we understand that there are days when toddlers do not grow and need fewer calories to live. These are the days when they are practicing what I term "eating air". They take a few bites or none, and the rest of the food is used as missiles. Then there are the days when they grow a ton and need lots of calories, so they eat and eat. Parents rejoice. This is short-lived, however, and kids quickly revert to an "all food is poison" mentality. Parents stress. Don't fret, here's help:

Don't Feed with Fear

- Parents fear malnutrition, middle of the night hunger, dehydration, being judged by friends and family members, and guilt. Fear alone leads parents to offer crackers, chips, cereals, and other white foods just to make sure their kids eat something. Toddlers scarf down the junk and the parents sigh with relief. When kids are not hungry, they don't eat what is served at dinner, but they will still eat junk food all day, any day.

Pro Tip:
A toddler refusing fruits/veggies/protein but eating crackers or cereal is not an indication of hunger. It is only an indication that they will eat a cracker at any time.

Don't Create Picky Eaters.

- If this pattern continues, the toddler, who is smarter than you think, begins to associate not eating his food with the right to get anything he pleases. This is when picky eating develops. Thus, suddenly, dinner becomes a buffet service. Who wants to do that every night at dinnertime?? *This is what should be feared: the buffet service, not the toddler.*

Got Too Much Milk?

- The traditional teaching is that after one year old, kids need to drink milk several times a day. The majority of toddlers I see in clinic drink 3-4 bottles/cups of milk a day AND they eat cheese, yogurt, butter, and some more cheese. I am not condemning dairy, but our kids eat and drink way too much. This delicious white food breaks down into lactose (a sugar) and casein which when digested it acts like a mild opiate. Anyone's kids addicted to their bottle of milk? The natural sugar in milk trains taste buds for sweets and carbs and the casein leaves them wanting more milk and cheese. Thus, vegetables get chucked at your head!

Pro Tip:
Decrease your child's milk intake to no more than 10 oz a day and allow for only one other serving of dairy per day.

Sit Down Please!

- Toddlers need to sit at the table. No roaming around with food. If they take a few bites and then they need to do a lap before returning to the table, so be it. They have the attention span of a goldfish. Again, food and drink are consumed only at the table.

Turn it Off!

- This may sound familiar but absolutely NO TV, NO iPads, and NO electronics at the table. A common misconception is that distraction equals better eating. Nope. Studies done on this exact topic show that kids who eat with the electronics off eat more veggies than those indulging in screen time at dinner. Eating in front of screens leads to weight issues in adolescence. Don't start habits that will be hard to break.

Beware of Portion Size.

- They need to be served the same dinner as the parents with an appropriate portion size. On average, portion size is one tablespoon per year of age. So, an 18-month-old should get 1.5 tablespoons of chicken, 1.5 tablespoons of mashed potatoes, and 1.5 tablespoons of green peas. Include a glass of milk or water.

Early Dinner Is Not an Excuse for Crappy Meals.

- If a toddler eats before the parents get home from work, use leftovers from the night before as their meal. Do not give them a hot dog and tater tots because they must eat early. So many times, parents eat amazing meals such as salmon, roasted potatoes, salad or baked veggies and the kids get processed nuggets, mac and cheese from a box, or hot dogs. Don't get me wrong, a hot dog at a cookout is no big deal. I am talking about incorporating them into the weekly meal plan. I know many will be upset by this tidbit because their hot dogs are all beef and organic. But do you eat hot dogs as your regular meal as an adult? If no, why not? If yes, then we might need to discuss *your* eating habits.

Do Not Cater to Children and Prepare Only What They Will Eat.

- Create one healthy meal for all and have a side of fruit or veggies that's a sure thing, for the questionable nights. This way all the food is on the table from the beginning. No one should be getting up to get something else when the child refuses to eat the meal. Every time a parent gets up to get the child another option to eat, the child learns that it pays not to eat what's in front of her. And so, "Parent Training" begins.

25% of the Meal is Used by the Brain [1]

- Toddler body growth may slow down, but brain growth is at its peak. For a brain to develop properly, it needs good, wholesome nutrition. The food you are serving them now will impact how they perform in elementary school. Processed food at this age is a thing to fear. Sugar in repeated doses interferes with brain development. More on this later.

Processed Foods Contribute to the Development of Chronic Disease

- There is a strong link between food and disorders of childhood and adolescence. Many of you have wondered about the "over-diagnosis" of ADHD in school children. How many of you have contemplated the over-indulgence of processed foods in toddler years as a root cause of the rise of ADHD in school kids?? How about anxiety, behavior issues, asthma, eczema, etc.? Yes, there are genetic components and environmental factors, but diet is a critical element for brain and body development. Avoid easy processed foods, as these can cause inflammation.

Other Things to Consider:

Be careful with snacks before dinner. There are so many different snack times, we don't even notice them. They have become like background noise. Examples:

- Snacks before kids are picked up from childcare, which is often close to mealtime

- Treats while shopping

- Sampling food at the grocery store

- Nibbles in the car, like fruit pouches

- Older siblings sneaking goodies to younger ones

- Snacks don't always appear as crackers; they can include milk, juice, yogurt, etc. I would love for all snacks to be a fruit/veggie/protein, but in the real world this is not the case the majority of the time.

Pro Tip:
No food of any kind two hours before and two hours after dinner.

OLDER CHILDREN

As Kids Continue to Grow, So Should Your Expectations of Them.

- Respect is vital. Children must sit at the table and show respect at all times. Do not tolerate, "I hate this," "This is disgusting," "Gross," "I am not eating this." (or other rude comments, complaints, or refusal). As all who prepare dinner know it takes a lot of thinking and planning to create the dinner meal. Do not allow disrespect at your table. If rude words are uttered, the child should be immediately excused from the table and they can get ready for bed. No snacks, no milk, nothing. I promise you; this will only happen a time or two. The message will be very clear without words needed.

- I have had to implement this in my house for two individuals *once*. Message was received by *all*. It was hard. I wanted to cry. I was worried that the two characters in question would starve to death. I quickly realized that it was 10 hours until breakfast; all would be okay. I do not tolerate impoliteness when I have worked so hard for the well-being of my family. Neither should you.

Eating is a romantic journey

- When children sit down at the table, we put food in front of them and they often reject it. Could it be that they missed the journey?

- When we as adults sit down to eat, it is the finale in our food romance. At first, we think and plan the meal. Then we touch, smell, and select the right foods at the store. At home we chop, mix, and feel the various ingredients, getting to know them better. The sizzling on the stove is an exciting sound announcing dinner is about to be ready. Aromas fill the kitchen as we dress the plates with various protein and veggie accessories. And when we finally sit down to eat, we don't just savor the food, but we taste the entire romantic journey.

- Allow the kids to join you on this food experience.

Have Kids Help with Shopping:

- They should be able to pick veggies and fruits at the store.

- You can do the color game (find a vegetable resembling a green stick), the alphabet game (find a fruit that starts with the letter O), and so on.

- Kids can choose produce, including peppers, cucumbers, carrots, oranges, apples, potatoes.

- Get excited about their efforts and teach them how to pick fruits and veggies to your liking.

- When kids get good at this, your shopping time will be cut by 25%. Trust me, I've done it! When the teens start driving, they will be able to help you with food shopping. Start now and you will thank me later.

- Don't be afraid to leave unwanted produce or kid-picked junk food items at the checkout counter.

- Bottom line: have them touch the veggies and be responsible for getting the family's food.

- If you have the time, energy, and space to grow a vegetable garden, go for it. Many studies link homegrown veggie gardens with improved childhood eating.

Let Kids Help in the Kitchen

0 TO 18 MONTHS

- Play with Tupperware, pots, pans, wooden spoons, and non-breakable dishes.

18 MONTHS TO 3 YEARS

- Wash veggies.
- Tear up greens.
- Put dry ingredients into bowls.
- Stir things.
- Rinse fruits and veggies.
- Scrub carrots and potatoes.
- Pick herbs off stems.
- Sprinkle herbs/salt/pepper.

- Mash veggies.

- Brush pastry or chicken with olive oil.

- Place silverware and non-breakables in the dishwasher, even though it's willy-nilly.

4 TO 5 YEARS OLD

- Cut things with a plastic knife.

- Peel fruits/veggies.

- Grate cheese and carrots and zest lemons.

- Juice lemons and limes.

- Crack eggs.

- Mix eggs.

- Mix dry goods for baking.

- Scoop meatballs with ice cream scooper.

- Scoop melons.

- Measure ingredients and spices.

- Mix salads with washed bare hands.

- Mix veggies for roasting.

- Arrange veggies for roasting.

6 TO 9 YEARS OLD

- Use garlic press, can opener, and grater.

- Form patties.

- Use a hand mixer.

- Whisk things.

- Use a paring knife.

- Cook at the stove, especially if you have an induction cooktop.

- Scrape mixer bowl.
- Slice bread.
- Grease baking pan.
- Roll dough.
- Put batter into muffin tray.
- Load and unload the dishwasher.

TEENS

- If you start cooking with your kids from an early age, there will be less complaining.
- If you ban electronics while you are cooking, they will help you.
- They may act like guests in your house, but they are members of your working community. These are skills they need to have when they move out, otherwise they will be lost in the world of fast food and convenience living.
- Kids who help in the kitchen eat a more varied diet than those who don't.
- Teenagers can cook, they just prefer someone do it for them.

A FEW MORE WORDS OF WISDOM:

- Serving veggies or salad before the rest of the meal increases veggie consumption by 40%.
- Never make the child finish what is on the plate.
- Never force-feed children.
- It is the parents' job to create what the meal is, when the meal is eaten, and where the meal is eaten.
- It is up to the child to decide how much to eat.

> **Pro Tip:**
> *For 24 hours, write down everything that goes in your child's mouth. When we start paying attention to the snack culture in our homes, interesting things are discovered. Snacks are one of the main reasons toddlers and kids who purportedly "eat nothing" are overweight. The calories are coming from somewhere.*

Final Note:

There are kids with oral/sensory aversion, sensory integration issues, and a true pathology to eating. These topics need to be addressed with a pediatrician and appropriate referrals need to be made. The sooner a therapist is engaged to deal with children's behavior/eating issues, the more likely those problems will be corrected.

When dealing with a stubborn child take 5 deep breaths and remember this: calling your child a "picky eater" simply reinforces the label for both of you. We parent according to labels. Children rise up to meet the expectations we set for them.

For my mega list of shopping items from Costco, Walmart, Trader Joe's, Target, Aldi, etc. scan the code for my book resources page.

3

You Can Teach Old Buds New Tricks

Retraining Taste Buds Leads to Healthy Eating

One does not undertake the mission of changing a family's eating habits without a generous dose of creativity, patience, and, most importantly, persistence. Our smoothie saga exemplifies the trials and tribulations involved in retraining the taste buds of marginally functioning small humans. The only way I could get them to drink smoothies initially was to essentially create milkshakes under the guise of a "protein shake". Our early test samples included milk, ice cream, and whatever fruit I could sneak in. I quickly realized I could secretly add more fruits, vegetables, and supplements without them suspecting a thing. This slowly evolved into adding a litany of healthier items to the drink until my evil genius plan was ultimately foiled. I overshot the mark the day I added kale, seaweed powder, beets, and leftovers from dinner; an all-out smoothie strike ensued. My husband is now in charge of the smoothies. We win some and we lose some.

Cells within taste buds generally live for ten to fourteen days. About one-third of taste bud cells die every 30 days, meaning that after 90 days we may have an entirely new set of taste bud cells. Because of this, we can train our taste buds to appreciate new flavors, to dislike intense sweetness/saltiness, and to enjoy foods that were once not appealing. Another interesting fact: companies that manufacture items we call food spend millions of dollars finding the right combination of chemicals to put into these food items to make us crave them longer, think about them often, and buy them more frequently. When was the last time you ate only one Lays Potato Chip? When that last Dorito is gone, do you look inside the bag in desperation? Mother Nature puts only one ingredient into each food she makes. Thus, when our taste buds are constantly bombarded and romanced by fancy chemicals in our food, it becomes difficult for us to really enjoy and appreciate real foods, such as broccoli, grapes, and spinach. A study by Jennifer Poti found that >75% of the foods Americans purchased from grocery stores is moderately or highly processed. [1] That means, the majority of the time, we are eating chemical experiments.

So how do you train taste buds to enjoy healthy foods?

FOOD

Bagels, pancakes, waffles, wraps, cereal, pasta, crackers, pretzels, cookies, and bread contain white flour, sugar, and a variety of other ingredients which cause them to have a high glycemic index. The body converts white flour into sugar, spiking blood sugar levels and causing insulin to rise quickly. When insulin rises too much and too fast, it shoves sugar into fat cells, the kind of fat cells the body has a difficult time accessing. Once sugar is pushed into fat cells, the blood sugar drops, leaving us hungry, cranky, fatigued, headachy, and craving more white flour and more sugar.

- Swap white flour products for high fiber foods that have whole wheat, brown rice, or oats as the first ingredient. The more fiber a product has, the more slowly it gets released into the bloodstream as sugar, which results in fewer cravings, longer times between meals, less fatigue, and fewer headaches.

- Look for at least three grams of fiber per serving. Foods should contain 12 to 15 percent of daily fiber requirement per serving. More than 15 percent is ideal (*Figure 1*).

Figure 1

Nutrition Facts

Serving Size 2 slices (68 g)
Servings Per Container 7

Amount Per Serving

Calories 190	**Calories from Fat 25**
	Calories From Saturated Fat 0

% Daily Value*

Total Fat 3g	**5%**
Saturated Fat 0g	**0%**
Trans Fat 0g	
Cholesterol 0mg	**0%**
Sodium 280mg	**12%**
Total Carbohydrate 38g	**13%**
Dietary Fiber 7g	➡ **28%**
Sugars 4g ⬆	
Protein 3g	**6%**
Vitamin A	**0%**
Vitamin C	**0%**
Calcium	**8%**
Iron	**15%**

- For non-plant eaters, start small. Place one grape or one slice of cucumber on a plate. Aim at having 1 fruit or 1 vegetable bite on the plate at each meal. Kids eat with their eyes first. Small amounts are doable. Do not make a big deal about it. Kids often need to be exposed to the same food over 21 times before they try it. It's ok!

- For lots of great ideas on food and snack substitutions, see the snack chapter next.

DRINKS

The biggest saboteurs of waistlines, harbingers of invisible sugar, and underrecognized suppressors of the immune system are drinks. They also contain unnecessary amounts of caffeine and food coloring. The beverage industry has tricked us into believing that our athletic performance will suffer without sports drinks. We fear that our children will perish from severe electrolyte imbalances if they play youth soccer without a sports drink. The TV has also convinced us that we will only have fun with a soda in our hand. Lastly, we shouldn't even consider jumping on a skateboard or dirt bike without that caffeinated drink which claims to give us wings.

Sadly, the marketing has blinded us to that fact that the beverage industry makes billions of dollars at the cost of our children's health. Based on multiple studies over the years, sugared drinks are the leading cause of obesity in children and teens.

RECOMMENDATIONS:

- Gradually decrease your daily intake of juice, soda, sports drinks, and sweet tea, the goal being none.
- Stop buying juice (yes even 100% juice, organic juice, orange juice, and apple juice).
- Try seltzer water infused with different pureed fruits.
- Buy a fruit infuser water bottle and mix and match flavors.
- Make OJ or lemonade at home from real fruit. This way the juice will be full of fiber, vitamins, and minerals.
- Watermelon slushie: watermelon + ice + blender
- Water and various milk varieties are ideal drinks. But beware that too much milk of any kind can sabotage the taste buds.

DRINK DILUTION SOLUTION:

If the whining in your house is simply too much, or you and your kids somehow cannot tolerate the taste of water, do a gradual dilution of sweet beverages. Here is the technique:

- Add water to the juice, sports drinks, or sweet tea. Start with a small amount and gradually add more and more until everything but the water is gone. If you bring any of these drinks into your home, begin the dilution immediately in the original bottle while unloading groceries. Add 1 ounce of water to the container of juice. Next time add 2 ounces of water to the juice bottle, and so on until it's mostly water. Thus, all unhealthy drinks are already diluted before anyone is the wiser.

- Three months from now when you and your family drink a regular sports drink, a glass of sweet tea, or a glass of juice, your taste buds will be shocked by the sweetness and your cravings will be significantly reduced.

ProTip:
White flour and sugar are highly addictive. The receptors in our brains react the same way to these foods as they would to drugs like cocaine or nicotine. The reward centers in our brains becomes less affected by these foods over time, so our brains crave larger and larger quantities in order to be satisfied. This leads to food cravings and binge eating.

At least 5 times a week offer a new food to try. Even if it's just one bite.

For my mega list of shopping items from Costco, Walmart, Trader Joe's, Target, Aldi, etc. scan the code.

4
Don't Kale My Vibe
How to get kids and husbands to eat more plants

Y'all have no idea how long I have tried to get my husband to eat more plants. Perhaps 23 years, but who's counting? Anywhoozle, several months ago I was out of town with the kids and John was at home on call. He randomly stumbled upon the documentary "The Game Changers". In this movie, plants are touted as the secret to a great physique, power in the gym, and better and longer erections. Guess who became a vegan for 5 days? Who knew that the secret to getting him to eat more plants, was hiding in the male sexual organ? He is no longer vegan, but he is counting and optimizing his plant points! I take my wins anyway I can.

I am certain we all know that we should eat more plants. In case you need a little refresher, plants are filled with vitamins, minerals, proteins, fats, and antioxidants which in turn power up our immune system, plump our skin, help us breathe easier, poop regularly, and have less boogers.

In his pivotal book *Fiber Fueled*, Dr Will Bulsiewicz explains, "Though food technology continues to progress, and we have more availability, the diversity in our diet is plummeting. As diversity of plants in our diets has decreased, chronic disease has increased."

For example

- 400,000 varieties of plants on earth
- 300,000 varieties are edible plants
- 200 species are eaten around the world

- 3 crops make 60% of the American diet
  - The 3 crops - corn, soybean, wheat

Not good my friends. We must be better. It doesn't mean you have to be vegan, it simply means we need to eat more plants. But how do we get kids to eat more plants?

In January 2021, inspired by @theguthealthmd, I launched an Instagram campaign to get kids to experiment with more plants - The Plant Point Challenge. Kids loved it and the adults wanted to be included as well. It was a smashing success. Here is how to get your family to enjoy more plants:

PLANT POINTS:

Things that count toward plant points:
- 1 point for each unique plant in your dish
  - So, 1 point for each fruit, veggie, dried fruit, quinoa, rice, grits, barley, millet, nuts, seeds, beans, hemp hearts, chia seeds
- Powdered plants such as kale, spinach, arugula, and beets count
- 1 point for nut milks
- Fresh herbs count. Dried herbs do not. (Though they are amazing)
- 1 bite of a plant counts

Things that DO NOT count toward your points:
- Wheat in a cracker
- Oats in a store-bought granola bar
- Strawberries in jelly or in Poptarts
- Fruit gummies, fruit roll up
- Store bought juice
- Maple syrup or honey

How to score your points per day:

Plant Point Scoring System			
Adults/Teens		Kids 1+	
Points	Plant Level	Points	Plant Level
1-21	Rookie	1-10	Beginner
21-24	Star	10-15	Up 'N Comer
24-28	Hero	15-20	Pro
28+	Hall of Fame	20+	Legend

Some examples for plant points with your meals:

Breakfast - Smoothie: 7 Plant Points

Oats(1), water, strawberries (1), cherries(1), mangoes(1), hemp hearts(1), Truvani plant based protein powder, honey, dates(1), spirulina(1)

Lunch - Salad & Homemade Mexican Burger: 12 Plant Points

Bib lettuce(1), red lettuce(1), red pepper(1), radish(1), olives(1), cucumbers(1), scallions(1), sheep feta, ground turkey, corn(1), beans(1), tomatoes(1), onions(1), fresh garlic(1)

Get your kids involved. Make it a family challenge each day, winner gets out of dish duty (this was a huge incentive for my tribe). Reset your gut! Your immune system will thank you.

When starting on your wellness journey aim for a minimum of 5 plant points a day.

For my mega list of shopping items from Costco, Walmart, Trader Joe's, Target, Aldi, etc. scan the code for my book resources page.

5

Snack Shark Attack

Navigating the dangerous waters of snack time

There was a time when I could basically get my kids to walk on hot coals for the promise of goldfish crackers. They should really just be called Goldfish Crack because millions of little addicts have been created world-over by their dealer parents distributing this tiny treat. I would pack the jumbo Goldfish chest from Costco into the car and feel the guilt of driving this much "product" over state lines. My first attempt to break the addiction involved purchasing the small snack packs of Goldfish and peddling them off for the promise of good behavior; but I still had all 3 kids jonesing for a fix. Ultimately, going cold turkey on the orange narcotic was the only way to solve my dilemma. Without the contraband in the house my alternative snack options were progressively accepted and we have now been "clean" for over 4 years!

Who is exhausted by the word "snack"? It seems like our kids are constantly shouting this word at us in hopes of receiving something sweet or processed. And this goes on all day, sunrise to sunset. Fun fact: snacking did not become popular until the 1950s, at which time it became the internationally known symbol of American life. In the economic boom succeeding World War II, processed foods and packaged snacks were marketed as high-quality and healthy. These innovations became popular because they took the drudgery out of homemaking. The stage was set.

In the 1980s snack foods exploded and packaged foods saturated our lives. Since then, we have been swimming in a sea of easily accessible, ready-made, terribly unhealthy snack food. Our kids have become the hungry sharks looking for a quick fix, and we have been more than willing to bait them by opening a package rather than peeling a fruit. Here are some healthier suggestions to satisfy the snack sharks.

FRUITS AND VEGGIES

Always offer a fruit or veggie snack as the first option

- Red pepper slices can replace chips.
- Grapes are a better choice than granola bars.
- Choose blueberries rather than fruit gummies.
- Orange slices provide more nutrients than juice.
- Carrot sticks with ranch dip
- Apple slices with nut butter
- Yogurt with fruit and granola
- Strawberries dipped in a yogurt or avocado cocoa dip
- Raspberries or carrot sticks are a great pre-dinner snack
- Smoothies
- Watermelon makes for a great desert
- Celery Ant Logs – celery, organic peanut butter, raisins
- Frozen grapes, peas, orange slices
- Nice Cream – made from frozen fruits and veggies
- Pickles
- Olives
- Salsa
- Good Foods or Kirkland brand avocado mash. These come in individual cups at Costco
- Hummus (Costco - individual size packs)

> **Pro Tip**
> Kids must eat a fruit or veggie before any packaged snack like pretzels,
> popcorn, or cheese sticks. If they refuse the healthy option, then they are
> not hungry. The end!

Eating something that comes directly from nature teaches children to fill their bellies with nutritious snacks rather than something less healthy from a package. This way, they fill themselves up with fruits and veggies and you won't have to continuously argue with them about too much junk food. This rule has also created a yes culture in our home. May I have popcorn? Yes, after you eat an apple. I'm still hungry, may I have pretzels? Yes, after you eat some carrots.

PACKAGED SNACKS WITH REAL INGREDIENTS.

Slowly finish what you have in your pantry and bring in new snacks that are less processed. You must be able to read all the ingredient to eat it. If you struggle pronouncing one of the ingredients or you must Google it, the snack is too processed. Put it back.

Good Snack Choices

- Siete chips
- Popcorn – Simply Popcorn
- Made Good Granola Bars or Granola Bites
- Lara Bars
- Homemade trail mix
- Crackers – Simple Mills, Back to Nature
- Banana plantain chips
- Crunchmaster Multi-Seed Olive Oil & Rosemary crackers
- Late July sea salt tortilla chips or potato chips

- Hippeas white cheddar chickpea snacks

- From the Ground Up cauliflower stars

- Turkey roll-up (buy Boars Head Simplicity or Fresh Fields) with cheese slice in the middle**

- Nuts and seeds (if age-appropriate) - aim for raw or simply roasted

- Rice cake with almond butter, sliced banana, a sprinkle of cinnamon

- Hard-boiled egg with Everything but the Bagel seasoning from Trader Joe's (also at Costco)

- Granola - Purely Elizabeth granola

- Applegate pepperoni with cheese and crackers

- Charcuterie platter**

**Refer to Chapter 12, "Where's the Beef" for more information

---

Pro Tip:
Fruits and veggies cut up and sitting on the counter disappear within 30 minutes. Fruits and veggies sitting in the fridge, even ready to eat, will remain untouched and grow mold.

At least 5 days per week, have a mix of fruits & veggies sitting on the counter.

For my mega list of shopping items from Costco, Walmart, Trader Joe's, Target, Aldi, etc. scan the code for my book resources page.

6

No Pop-Tart Party Here

Make Breakfast the Meal of Champions

Ok, full disclosure here. We were a Pop-Tart/Toaster Strudel with a side of Cinnamon Toast Crunch kind of family for many years. You can imagine the horror we initially faced when replacing those dandies with fruits, homemade oatmeal, and smoothies. It's tough enough just getting them to put shoes on the right feet much less battle them over breakfast options. But it's the change that's hard and kids will settle into their new reality. Our kids now get out of bed and ask for their smoothies!

The Biggest Issues with Breakfast are as Follows:

- Kids want sugar in the form of cereal, waffles, bagels, toast, pancakes, granola bars, etc.

- These white foods are easy breakfast options.

- A high carbohydrate meal, with or without sugar, lasts in the body only 30-45 minutes, leading to a sugar crash as the child begins their morning learning. This results in: inattention, anxiety, mood swings, tantrums, memory issues, etc.

> **ProTip:**
> The brain utilizes 25% of the food, vitamins, and minerals from a meal.
> Therefore, if you start your children's day with a high carbohydrate and/
> or high sugar meal, their brains will be fueled by sugar. This results in
> behavior issues.

Teens often complain of nausea, not being hungry, and not having enough time for breakfast. **Here are some easy fixes:**

- Not enough time:
    - Employ better time management tools in the morning.
    - Go to sleep earlier to have more time in the morning.
    - Don't snooze the alarm 57 times.
- Nausea:
    - No eating late at night. Stop eating 2 hours before bed.
    - No fast food for dinner.
- Not hungry:
    - This is legit. Who wants to eat a full meal at 6:00am? Having a good school-friendly snack with fat/protein/plants during the morning blocks can solve this problem.

Here are a few breakfast options for a healthy immune system and an attentive brain. These can help the entire family get the day started on the right foot.

- Toast with avocado and "Everything but the Bagel" seasoning
- Eggs and nitrite-free bacon**
- Nitrite free chicken sausage from the butcher**
- Homemade waffles previously cooked and frozen can be defrosted in the toaster and smeared with nut butter and sliced bananas or topped with berries.

- Whole grain toast with nut butters, banana slices, or a drizzle of honey

- Seeded crackers, cream cheese, smoked salmon

- Smoothies

- Dinner leftovers. Yes, this can be breakfast. The leftovers don't know that they should be only eaten at 6:00 p.m.

- Homemade oatmeal. Don't even consider the packets! Try overnight oatmeal.

- Scrambled eggs with spinach

- Charcuterie platter**

- Homemade granola with plant-based milk or yogurt and berries

- Nuts and berries

- PB & J layered with fruits

- Chia pudding

** Refer to Chapter 12, "Where's the Beef" for more information

Make breakfast a meal of champions at least 5 days per week.

For my mega list of shopping items from Costco, Walmart, Trader Joe's, Target, Aldi, etc. scan the code.

7

Let 'Em Steal Your Lucky Charms
The Great Cereal Debate

American breakfast cereals hold some sort of mystical taste bud hijacking power over us. When I was a kid, we were defined by our trademark cereal. I was an Apple Jacks girl, my husband was a Cap'n Crunch man, and all my kids worshipped Cinnamon Toast Crunch. But the ultimate power of cereal is evident in a story from my husband, John's, childhood. One summer night John's mom finally agreed to buy him a box of Cap'n Crunch, which, until that time, he had only sampled at friends' houses and camp. Additionally, he was allowed to have a friend, whom we will call George, spend the night. With his happiness now complete, John woke up the next morning and enthusiastically bounded down the stairs to enjoy his first bowl of the scrumptious, crunchy delight. As he rounded the corner, the macabre scene at the breakfast table nearly made him faint. George had awakened early and eaten the entire box of Cap'n Crunch in one sitting!

Unimpressed with this feat of gluttony, but feeling guilt over his new hatred of George, John proceeded to his Catholic school later that week when confessions were on the agenda. He entered the confessional and extolled the horrors of the recent cereal incident to the forgiving priest. With a smile on his face, the priest explained to John that no, he would not be going to hell for his new desire to kill George and that he probably should focus a bit less on cereal. I am proud to say that John has finally kicked the habit.

In terms of nutrition, I am opposed to all store-bought cereals. There is really no such thing as healthy cereal. Sugar is an obvious reason. Even if the cereal claims to be low in sugar, the carbohydrates are converted directly into sugar. There are several other culprits as well.

FOOD COLORING

- There are now hundreds of studies showing the link between food coloring and children's behavior.[1]
- To better understand how food coloring affects children, watch this 1 min Pediatrics Video by scanning the QR code with your phone.

https://youtu.be/mGJl4eZjPpw

FIBER

- Not all fiber is created equal.
- The fiber in many cereals is full of phytates, substances that can bind up essential vitamins and nutrients and take them out of the body leading to deficiencies.
- Some fiber comes from wood pulp. Yummy.

VITAMINS

How many ads have you seen about cereal providing a complete breakfast? The companies suggest that the box in front of you has all the vitamins and minerals needed to grow. Really??

Mother Nature understands only vitamins and minerals that come from plants, eggs, meats, and whole foods, not the chemicals created in a lab. Synthetic vitamins are made by scientists and added to garbage to give us the impression of food. Generally, the body does not understand things like "tocopherols" (synthetic Vitamin E).

Many parents know not to buy multivitamins such as Flintstones because they are full or garbage, food coloring, sugar and synthetic ingredients. For those of you who didn't know, now you do! That's okay. It took me a while to learn this as well. Many parents scour the nutrition labels of vitamins making sure they come from a natural source. Yet many of those same parents feed their kids food with added synthetic vitamins made from who knows what. These fake vitamins get excreted by the body to make very expensive urine. Lastly, some of these manufactured vitamins can become harmful in large quantities.

SO, WHAT IS A PARENT TO DO?

Check out the breakfast chapter. It contains lots of ideas of breakfasts made from real foods. I know everyone is busy. But let's make better food choices now and avoid chronic disease later. Undoing the damage is a lot harder, more expensive, and much more time consuming.

- If you must buy foods in a package or container, make sure they don't contain fake vitamins.
- Milk substitutes are notorious for synthetics.
- Baby cereals claim to improve your baby's iron levels but they contain an added side of arsenic.

My Agenda Here: Get Rid of Cereals Altogether.

Avoid cereal 5 days a week, especially on school days.

For my mega list of shopping items from Costco, Walmart, Trader Joe's, Target, Aldi, etc. scan the code for my book resources page.

8

A Whopper of a Bad Decision

Fast Food Alternatives

Let me create the scenario: It's Monday night and I'm in my minivan picking up the last child from an endless litany of activities. It's 8:00 PM and no one has eaten. On the way home, the Burger King drive through seemed to be the only logical option as every kid loves chicken cooked in a cesspool of oils. Once I realized the error of my ways, I took the next logical step and changed our Monday night fast food to Subway as a "healthier choice". Then I was informed their bread was created from the same chemical used to make yoga mats. Thanks Food Babe! Thus, I arrived at our current technique for busy nights, I made sandwiches for the car or put leftovers in a thermos. Decreasing our activities was also a viable option, but let's not get too carried away here.

Should you avoid fast food? Is all fast food bad? You need to be knowledgeable about what goes into the food to make that decision. Be careful though, marketing in this industry is very effective. There are healthy fast-food choices, but they are few and far between. Always ask to see the ingredients to make an educated decision. Let's review some ingredients.

Here is a list of ingredients from Chik-Fil-A directly from their website:

CHICKEN NUGGETS:

Chicken (boneless, skinless chicken breast meat nuggets, salt, <u>monosodium glutamate</u>, sugar, spices, paprika, enriched bleached flour [with malted barley flour, niacin, iron, thiamine mononitrate, riboflavin, folic acid], sugar, salt, <u>monosodium glutamate</u>, nonfat milk, leavening [baking soda, sodium aluminum phosphate, monocalcium phosphate], spice, <u>soybean oil</u>, color [paprika], pasteurized nonfat milk, pasteurized egg, fully refined peanut oil [with <u>dimethylpolysiloxane</u> {an anti-foam agent} added]).

Comparison of McDonald's **French Fries** Ingredients U.S. vs U.K.

McDonalds French Fries Ingredients	
United States	**United Kingdom**
Potatoes, Vegetable Oil (Canola Oil, <u>Hydrogenated Soybean Oil</u>, Natural Beef Flavor [Wheat and milk derivatives], Citric Acid [preservative]), Dextrose, <u>Sodium Acid Pyrophosphate</u> (maintain color), Salt. Prepared in Vegetable Oil (Canola Oil, Corn Oil, <u>Soybean Oil</u>, <u>Hydrogenated Soybean Oil</u> with TBHQ and Citric Acid added to preserve freshness. <u>Dimethylpolysiloxane</u> added as an antifoaming agent	Potatoes, Vegetable Oil (Sunflower, Rapeseed), Dextrose (only added at beginning of season). Prepared in the restaurants using a non-hydrogenated vegetable oil. Salt is added after cooking. (Created by Food Babe)

A QUICK SUMMARY TO KEEP IT SIMPLE:

Monosodium Glutamate (MSG)

- Studies on eating MSG have shown MSG to cause headaches, chest tightness, flushing, and muscle tightness in genetically susceptible people. [1]

- The "Chinese Restaurant Syndrome" is a real thing and is also known as the MSG symptom complex. These symptoms often include headache, skin flushing, and sweating in sensitive people after eating at a Chinese restaurant. [2]

- There is evidence that MSG induces the cell death of neurons. [3]

Soybean Oil: Heavily Processed and Refined

- In other words, many chemicals are used to turn soybeans into oil.

- Also, the majority of soybeans in the US are genetically modified, making it the crop with the highest levels of glyphosate, an herbicide and pesticide linked to Non-Hodgkin's lymphoma, Parkinson's disease, immune system problems and hypothyroidism. [4]

- It is also high in Omega-6, a contributor to chronic disease in elevated amounts.

Hydrogenated Soybean Oil

- Hydrogenated or partially hydrogenated means it is a trans-fat.

- Trans fats have been shown to cause heart disease and death.

- The FDA has mandated the removal of these from foods in 2018. [5]

- But beware, the FDA allows food with less than 0.5grams of trans fat per serving to claim "0" grams of trans fat on their labels. Thus, read ingredients and if you see partially hydrogenated or hydrogenated anything on the list, put it back.

Sodium Acid Pyrophosphate

- Has been shown to have toxic effects on blood cells and the immune system in rats. [6]

- There are no human studies to prove its safety, yet it is approved for general public consumption in the US.

Dimethylpolysiloxane, the Anti-Foaming Agent

- There is no research to show that this is safe in foods despite being approved by the FDA in 1998.

- At high temperatures, such as, let's say hot oil during frying, it degrades into formaldehyde, a known cancer-causing agent. [7]

- Moreover, this anti-foaming agent is banned in Europe, Australia and New Zealand. My question continues to be, if they can do it, why can't we?

Families occasionally want to eat out and make dinner easy and fun. Here is what you need to know:

Healthy Restaurant Options and Tips:

- Don't take your child to their favorite restaurant if they are not allowed to have their favorite food. That is setting them up for failure.

- Generally speaking, do not order food from the children's menu.

- Research the restaurant before you go and choose the meals everyone in your family will be eating so you do not have to spend much time looking at the menu.

- Most restaurants show ingredients on their websites; check these out first.

- Have your child be involved in picking out the meal so they don't' get frustrated.

- For families trying to avoid dairy and gluten without having celiac disease or anaphylaxis, don't worry about trace amounts of gluten and dairy. If a restaurant asks if your request is a preference or allergy related, you can say preference. Most restaurants cannot guarantee there is no cross contamination and therefore err on the side of caution.

ProTip
When traveling, pack whole foods in a cooler and load up on wholesome snacks. This will help minimize stops at fast food restaurants in the middle of nowhere. When fast food happens to good people, sub fruit for fries, skip the soda, get a salad, and omit the dressing. Avoid kids' meals.

There are plenty of restaurant options in various categories:

Rotisserie Chicken:

- Sides can include rice, quinoa, corn, beans, sweet potato fries, yuca, and/or salad.

Fresh Mexican:

- Corn tacos with chicken or beef, salsa and guacamole
- Rice bowls with beans and choice of meat, veggies, salsa, and guacamole
- Taco salads with meat, veggies, salsa and corn chips are also an option for kids willing to eat a salad.
- Sides include corn, beans, rice, veggies, chips, salsa.

Asian:

- Avoid chains and stick with local.
- Look for any type of stir fry or hibachi mixing rice, veggies, chicken, beef, pork, or shrimp.
- If you want to avoid gluten, ask for the sauce to be GF (like GF soy sauce).
- Noodle dishes that are made with GF noodles include vermicelli, cellophane noodles, rice noodles, Hanoi noodles soba noodles. Buckwheat, despite having the word wheat in it, is GF. Make sure they are 100% buckwheat as some cheaper restaurants will mix in wheat.
- Spring Rolls in rice paper, Sushi, Thai Curry.

American Fair:

- Grilled chicken, steak, fish, ribs, pulled pork, hamburger.
- Sides can include baked potato, sweet potato, green beans, corn, fruit, rice, quinoa, salad, beans, broccoli, and sweet potato fries.

- Chopped salad. Children may surprise you with eating a salad especially if it is "chopt". Small crunchy bites of lettuce are easier textures for children than soggy long greens. Let your children pick out their topping and their own dressing to make it a more fun experience.

Greek:

- Chicken, beef, or lamb skewers can be a fun way for kids to eat.

- Grape leaves (dolmades), souvlaki, roasted potatoes, grilled meats, chickpea salad

Mediterranean:

- Chicken, beef, lamb with sides of fresh veggies, and pita bread

If you can't avoid fast food, choose menu items with fewer than 5 ingredients.

For my mega list of shopping items from Costco, Walmart, Trader Joe's, Target, Aldi, etc. scan the code for my book resources page.

9
Don't Shop 'til You Drop!
Grocery Shopping Made Easier

One of the first steps in my journey toward healthier food choices was changing my grocery store habits. Not only did I spend quite a bit of time in the less healthy "middle" aisles, but I would always tend to buy the brand that I recognized (i.e., the brand that spent the most on marketing). When I began to look for different products, I was overwhelmed by the sheer number of choices - I mean how many gluten-free pastas does a store need? I would stand in the aisles and Google the product in an attempt to decipher the healthier brand. My breakthrough was realizing the power of 5 when reading labels. I would only buy a product if it had fewer than 5 ingredients. This drastically reduced the pool of eligible items to choose from and made me feel better about what I was putting into my family's bodies. And moreover, my grocery illiterate husband now uses the same rule to guide him through the store.

Healthy eating begins at the grocery store. If you shop with an unhealthy mindset, you will come home with subpar selections. If your kids are complaining throughout the grocery shopping experience about the food you buy and you cannot resist them, get a babysitter, and leave them home. It will still be cheaper than buying the junk your kids demand, trust me. Once the kids are compliant with the foods you choose, take them with you and have them help with selecting foods. Use the following tips to make the most of your grocery store ventures.

GROCERY STORE ATTACK PLAN

- Meal prep is the key to saving dollars and sanity. At the start of the week, make a list of dinners you wish to cook and create the shopping list accordingly.

- Make the list correlate with the order of your shopping. Group items from the same section together on the list. It makes shopping much faster and easier.

- Keep the list on the fridge and write down items as you run out of them. To be honest, I am terrible at this, but it's a work in progress.

- Never shop on an empty stomach.

- Beware of junk food sales. It's marketing and it works. I often hear people say in clinic, "I had to buy 5 packs of ice cream, cuz they had a buy two get three free sale."

- I love produce sales. Grocery stores often run specials on seasonal fruits and veggies. A sale here should attract your attention to in-season items which often contain the most nutrition.

- Shop first thing in the morning (before 9:00 a.m.) to avoid crowds and get the freshest produce.

- Grab perishable items from the back of the shelf. They are generally stacked oldest to freshest, oldest in the front, freshest in the back.

- Shop the perimeter: produce, dairy, bread, seafood, and meat can be found at the perimeter of the store, while everything else is consolidated in the center.

ProTip
Be okay with going to the store more than once or twice a week. When we try to avoid the grocery store for weeks at a time, we end up buying a lot of processed foods.

Aisles That Are Beneficial:

- Frozen fruits/veggies
- Baking/spices
- International section
- Bread
- Coffee/tea

Avoid the Following Aisles, Nothing Good Happens Here:

- Soda/juice
- Chips/crackers
- Cookies/chocolate
- Breakfast
- Salad dressing
- Wine

 Shop the perimeter! If you must venture into the middle, shop fewer than 5 aisles.

If you would like to come grocery shopping with me, join me on my channel - Ana-Maria Temple, MD YouTube

10

Old MacDonald Had an Organic Farm

Understanding the Importance of Organic Foods

I vividly remember standing in my kitchen being interrogated by my husband who was holding multiple grocery store receipts from the previous few months. There had been an expected increase in the grocery costs associated with buying higher quality organic foods and he felt we were pouring money down the drain. Listening to him drone on, I couldn't help but think about the fancy sports car he had purchased which sat in the garage most of the time and, of course, only consumed high octane, high-cost premium fuel. I calmly opined on the fact that it was rational to spend extra money on the high-quality gas in his beloved car but was a waste to spend extra money on food not covered in pesticides.
The result? He no longer owns a sports car and we enjoy the benefits of organic foods!

How important is it to eat organic foods? Is there science to support these claims or is it simply marketing? And what does the term organic even mean?

The label "organic" describes the way farmers grow and process fruits, vegetables, grains, dairy products and meat. In this chapter we will only focus on *plants.*

Organic practices *do not* permit the following:

- Synthetic fertilizers
- Sewage sludge as fertilizer
- Most synthetic pesticides for pest control
- Irradiation to preserve food or to eliminate disease or pests
- Genetic engineering (GMO), used to improve disease control or pest resistance or to improve crop yields
- Antibiotics or growth hormones for livestock

Organic practices *do* permit the following:

- Plant waste left on fields (green manure), livestock manure or compost to improve soil quality
- Plant rotation to preserve soil quality and to interrupt cycles of pests or disease
- Cover crops that prevent erosion when parcels of land are not in use and to plow into soil for improving soil quality
- Mulch to control weeds
- Predatory insects or insect traps to control pests
- Certain natural pesticides and a few synthetic pesticides approved for organic farming, used rarely and only as a last resort in coordination with a USDA organic certifying agent

The Different Organic Labels Explained

- **100 Percent Organic**: All ingredients present in the product are organic.
- **Organic**: At least 95 percent of the product's ingredients are organic.
- **Made with Organic Ingredients**: At least 75 percent of the product's ingredients are organic.
- **Organic Ingredients Noted on the Ingredients Statement**: Less

than 70 percent of the product's ingredients are organic, so the producer can only identify the specific organic ingredients on the product label. [1]

Are There Benefits to Organic Food?

- **Nutrients**. Studies have shown small to moderate increases in some nutrients in organic produce. The best evidence of a significant increase is in certain types of flavonoids which have antioxidant properties.

- **Pesticide Residue.** Compared with conventionally grown produce, organically grown produce has lower detectable levels of pesticide residue. Organic produce may have residue because of pesticides approved for organic farming or because of airborne pesticides from conventional farms. [2,3,4,5]

- **Toxic Metal**. Cadmium is a toxic chemical naturally found in soils and absorbed by plants. Studies have shown significantly lower cadmium levels in organic grains, though not in fruits and vegetables, when compared with conventionally grown crops. The lower cadmium levels in organic grains may be related to the ban on synthetic fertilizers in organic farming.

- **Bad news**. Unfortunately, recent reports have shed light on Heavy Metals in baby food and based on the 2021 congressional hearing, organic farms do not have to test their soils for heavy metals: lead, cadmium, arsenic, and mercury. Several studies and a congressional hearing found unacceptably high levels of toxic heavy metals in popular organic baby food and formula.

To get my complete guide on safe baby foods, go to my book resources page:

Medical Research Findings on Herbicides and

Pesticides:

- Farm workers on non-organic farms, have higher rates of cancer and increased rates of respiratory illnesses such as cough, asthma, COPD, seasonal allergies, etcetera, according to studies performed in 1997 and 2001. [6,7]

- Increased pesticide exposure in children of farm workers showed an increase in cancer rates, specifically, leukemia, neuroblastoma, Wilms' tumor, non-Hodgkin's lymphoma, brain cancer, colorectal cancer, and testicular cancer as found in 2 extensive literature reviews conducted in 1998 and 2007. [8,9,10]

- Organophosphate exposure (pesticides) measured by residue in children's urine, was shown to be linked to a one to two-fold increase in ADHD symptoms for children 8-15 years old.[11]

- Children exposed prenatally to pesticides and herbicides have lower scores for mental and motor development (study 2007), greater likelihood of behavioral issues (study 2006), decreased birth weight (study 2004), smaller head circumference (study 2004). [12,13,14,15,16]

- Kids exposed prenatally to pesticides were followed for 7 years and the exams showed an overall decrease in development and increase in behavioral issues at ages 2 years and 7 years. [17]

- A study in 2006 showed that urine levels of pesticides were dramatically reduced in children who were placed on an organic diet for just one week. [18]

Why Should We Change to Organic Products?

- Organic produce contains less pesticide residue than conventional produce. Levels of pesticides from exposure to conventional produce equals that seen in farm workers on non-organic farms. (see list of illnesses above)

- 80% of the pesticide/herbicide exposure to humans comes from produce. [19]

- Washing and peeling cannot completely remove the pesticide residues. [20]

- Pesticide-free is only addressing the pesticide part of the organic issue. You must also take this on faith. There are no inspection standards here.

- Organic farms are regularly inspected and must pass numerous tests to be certified and to keep their certification.

- Every time we choose organics we vote for the food with fewer chemicals, better farming, more crop rotations, and a more sustainable environment.

How to Choose Affordable Organic Produce

- Choose organic produce that is on the Dirty Dozen list, then move to the others. More than 98 percent of strawberries, spinach, peaches, nectarines, cherries, and apples tested positive for at least one pesticide residue according to the Environmental Working Group (EWG). As a general rule, the thinner the skin, the more likely it is that pesticides can leak through.

- Costco is the largest retailer of organic food. Affordable organic produce can be now found at Walmart, Aldi, Target, and other grocery store around the country.

- Eat fewer animal products and more fruits and vegetables.

- Shopping at farmers markets for items that are in season will reduce costs.

- Sign up with your community for Azure Standard. It is an organization that delivers affordable organic food to your neck of the woods.

- Join a co-op or Community Supported Agriculture (CSA) where customers buy shares of a farm's harvest in advance.

- Stop buying junk such as soda, Gatorade, juice, and Powerade and use the savings from these products to buy organic. Remember water is free.

- Replace snacks like Doritos, Cheetos, and cookies with healthier alternatives.

- Frozen fruits and veggies are cheaper than fresh ones.

- Meal prep: get as many uses as possible out of bulk items. For example, using carrots in several recipes in a week will reduce waste.

- Freeze stuff. Once you cut up fresh organic fruits and veggies for your meals, freeze the rest to use at a later time. I freeze leftovers such as mushrooms, zucchini, cauliflower, herbs. I use frozen veggies to make soups, smoothies, and casseroles. I add them to sauces or curry and mix them in burgers or sloppy joes, to name a few.

- Dehydrate fruits or veggies and turn them into snacks.

- Grow your own veggies. I recently invested in the Tower Garden and am currently growing 20 different veggies and herb

The Dirty Dozen		
(Buy these organic whenever possible)		
1. Strawberries	5. Spinach	9. Kale
2. Nectarines	6. Apples	10. Grapes
3. Peaches	7. Cherries	11. Pears
4. Tomatoes	8. Celery	12. Potatoes

The Clean 15		
(Consider non-organic if organic is unavailable)		
1. Avocados	6. Sweet peas	11. Broccoli
2. Sweet corn	7. Asparagus	12. Pineapple
3. Eggplant	8. Mushrooms	13. Cabbage
4. Onions	9. Cauliflower	14. Honeydew
5. Papaya	10. Cantaloupes	15. Kiwifruit

 Eat fewer than 5 nonorganic foods per day.

For my mega list of shopping items from Costco, Walmart, Trader Joe's, Target, Aldi, etc. scan the code.

11

So Many Fish in the Sea

What to Eat to Increase Omega-3s & Decrease Exposure to Mercury

They say it takes a village to raise a child but, in our case it took blatant deception about fish. Fish wasn't a popular meal in our house and was rejected outright by my youngest and pickiest eater. Our clever solution was to tell a mild white lie about mild white fish. Upon serving tilapia one night at dinner, my youngest questioned why the "chicken" looked different. Our explanation was, "This is specialized chicken from the town of Tilapia, Indiana and it tastes even better than regular chicken." We subsequently introduced "chicken" from the great cities of Mahi Mahi, Texas; Halibut, South Dakota; Grouper, Tennessee; and, of course, Cod, Rhode Island. Problem solved!

Fatty fish are a great source of Omega-3, an unsaturated fat that is critical to overall health. Our bodies cannot make sufficient Omega-3 and so depend on food sources for this healthy fat. Omega-3 is needed for...

Brain Development in Fetuses and Children

- The most rapid brain growth occurs in the uterus and in the first 2 years of life.

- Furthermore, the brain continues to grow and develop into our late twenties.

Nerve Connections

- These are constantly being regenerated.

- Nerve connections are responsible for enhancing focus, concentration, and memory.

- Check out this 1-minute video about how omega 3 increases the conduction of electrical impulses for a smarter and more efficient brain.

https://youtu.be/AJrSpYYCRZE

Omega-3s Prevent Chronic Disease By:

- Reducing colds, flu, and sore throats by enhancing the immune system [1,2]

- Reducing asthma symptoms [3]

- Decreasing menstrual cramps [4]

- Improving skin tightness and adjunct for healing eczema [5]

- Decreasing acne [6]

- Improving children's sleep [7]

- Decreasing risk of developing childhood type 1 diabetes [8]

- Relieving dry eyes [9]

- Enhancing child brain development [10]

- Improving symptoms of depression, anxiety, and ADHD [11,12,13,14]]

- Improving nonalcoholic fatty liver disease (yes this is on the rise in children) [15]
- Decreasing symptoms of arthritis and muscle aches [16]
- Improving heart health [17]
- Improving vision [18]

Nearly all demographics have too little fish in their diets. This includes:

- Pregnant women
- Nursing women
- Children
- Teenagers

Why the lack of fish? Because people are terrified of mercury. But who is really at risk? Children are especially vulnerable because in the first 1 to 6 months after birth, the pathways to process chemicals and toxins are immature. Fetuses and children undergo rapid brain growth and critical development of their nervous system. This growth puts them at high risk for complications from exposure. Developing fetuses may be seriously affected even though the mother shows no symptoms of mercury exposure. [19]

- **High Dose Effect**: mental retardation, cerebral palsy, and hearing loss
- **Low Dose Chronic Exposure Effect:** issues with motor function, information processing, memory, vocabulary, and attention

Fetal Effects

The fetus is at the highest risk of neurological effects due to developing nervous systems (four to five times more sensitive than adults).

Methyl mercury can cross the placenta and the blood-brain barrier.

Mercury is then concentrated in the brain of the fetus because the metal is absorbed quickly and is not excreted efficiently. [20,21]

Exposed fetuses may be born with symptoms resembling:

- Cerebral Palsy, spasticity, or other movement abnormalities
- Convulsions
- Visual problems
- Abnormal reflexes
- Delays in walking, talking, and lifelong learning difficulties.

How does mercury get into the environment?

- Coal burning plants
- Waste incinerators
- Industrial release from cement and metal producing plants
- Small scale gold mining
- Natural sources
- Disposal of latex paint, batteries, BP machines, compact fluorescent bulbs, skin lightening creams
- Dental fixtures and dental sealants
- Ethyl mercury in vaccines. This has been removed from children's vaccines since 2001. However, trace amounts can be found in the Tdap and in multidose flu vaccines. [22]
- Dental sealants. Two independent studies in 2006 showed no neurological effects in children 3 years old with sealants. [23]
- However, a recent study from 2018 showed a relationship between body burden of mercury from dental amalgams and ADHD. [24]

Here are some ways to get healthy Omega-3, DHA and EPA into your diet without being exposed to high levels of mercury.

Women of child-bearing age, nursing women, and young children may eat the following small fish two times per week: shrimp, salmon, and canned light tuna. Canned light tuna is very low in mercury and is not restricted.

For the rest, do not be afraid of fish; just choose wisely!

Other Sources of Omega-3

- Chia seeds: 3Tbsp = 4800 mg Omega-3

- Hemp Hearts: 3Tbsp = 3000mg Omega-3

- Flax Seed Powder: 2 Tbsp= 2800mg Omega-3

- Barlean's Flax Seed Oil is another great alternative that is sweet and flavorful, comes in berry and banana strawberry: 1 TBSP = 1000mg Omega-3.

- Walnuts: 1oz = 2654mg Omega-3

Best Choices - Eat 2 to 3 Servings Per Week		
Anchovy	Hake	Scallop
Atlantic Croaker	Herring	Shad
Atlantic Mackerel	Lobster, American and Spiny	Shrimp
Black Seabass	Mullet	Skate
Butterfish	Oyster	Smelt
Catfish	Pacific Chub Mackerel	Sole
Clam	Perch, Freshwater and Ocean	Squid
Cod	Pickerel	Tilapia

Crab	Plaice	Trout, Freshwater
Crawfish	Pollack	Tuna, Canned White (Includes Skipjack)
Flounder	Salmon	Whitefish
Haddock	Sardine	Whiting

Good Choices - Eat 1 Serving per Week

Blue fish	Monkfish	Striped Bass (Ocean)
Buffalo fish	Rockfish	Tilefish (Atlantic Ocean)
Carp	Sablefish	Tuna, Albacore White Tuna, Canned and Fresh/Frozen
Chilean Sea Bass, Patagonian Toothfish	Sheepshead	Tuna, Yellow Finn
Grouper	Snapper	Weakfish/Seatrout
Halibut	Spanish Mackerel	White Croaker/ Pacific Croaker
Mahi Mahi, Dolphinfish		

Choices to Avoid - Highest Mercury Levels

King mackerel	Shark	Tilefish (Gulf of Mexico)
Marlin	Swordfish	Tuna (Bigeye)
Orange Roughy		

Guide for Pregnant Women:

Pregnant women do **not** eat: Large fish like shark, swordfish, king mackerel, sea bass, albacore tuna, or tilefish.

Eat Omega-3-rich foods more than 5 times a week.

For my mega list of shopping items from Costco, Walmart, Trader Joe's, Target, Aldi, etc. scan the code for my book resources page.

12

Where's the Beef?

Understanding the Red Meat We Eat

When I got married, I never imagined my meat choices would become a source of spousal conflict. But I found myself once again standing in my kitchen defending the grocery bill and the marginal increase in cost to buy grass-fed hormone-free beef. He snarkily asked "Do they pet and massage the cows? Do they whisper sweet nothings in their ears? Do they sleep on memory foam mattresses?" My response was to have him watch the documentary Food Inc. I blissfully watched his horrified face as he began to understand the environmental, inhumane, and health issues of our beef industry. Not only did we drastically reduce our meat intake, but we also became very selective about the meat we do buy. Our ultimate goal is to be meat free, but I realize this transition is not a sprint; it's a marathon.

Should we have meat in our diets? I am a big believer in eating from all food groups, except for the "fast food group." That said, I do feel Americans eat too much meat. 50-75% of our plates should be filled with plants. Fun fact: The U.S. is the number one meat consumer in the world. Great, but when you do eat meat, how should you choose the best products?

The World Health Organization (WHO) classifies red meat as 2A, meaning it is possibly carcinogenic to humans. There is some evidence that there is an association between eating red meat and developing colon cancer.[1]

Red meat refers to all mammalian muscle meat, including beef, veal, pork, lamb, mutton, horse, and goat.

Understanding Meat Labels. These are the labels on meat you should pay attention to:

- American Grass-fed Association (AGA)
- Organic
- Animal Welfare Approved
- Certified Humane
- Certified Naturally Grown
- Global Partnership

American Grass-fed Association - The Best Choice

- Label: American Grass-fed Association Label
- Applies to cattle, bison, goats, and sheep.
- Diet: 100% fed from an open pasture
- Living conditions: Live only on open pastures with access to shelter
- Antibiotics/Hormones: None allowed
- Origin: U.S. born/raised

Organic - Second Best. The FDA puts fewer restrictions on organic meat compared to AGA certified meat.

- Diet: Blended grain and corn, mixed in with grazing on grass, diet free from synthetic herbicides, pesticides, or fertilizers, non-GMO feed
- Living: Some inconsistencies seen here, generally animals are not kept in confined spaces for long periods of time; ex: dairy cattle have to be on the pasture for at least 120 days of the year
- Antibiotics/Hormones: None allowed

Animal Welfare Approved (AWA): Most Rigorous Form of Labeling

- Animals raised outdoors on pasture

- No cages, crates, or tethers; no alterations to animals
- No hormones: antibiotics only given to sick animals
- Welfare-oriented slaughter guidelines
- Certification: Only given to family farms

Certified Humane:

- Diet: Animals raised outdoors on pasture
- Living: No cages, crates, or tethers; living conditions have meticulous restrictions to ensure animals live in natural conditions
- Antibiotics/Hormones: No hormones or antibiotics
- Other: Welfare-oriented slaughter guidelines
- Certification: Only given to family farms
- Diet: Standards are very similar to USDA Organic with tighter requirements for access to pasture; free from synthetic herbicides, pesticides, or fertilizers
- Antibiotics/Hormones: No hormones or antibiotics
- Difference: Audits are done by other Certified Naturally Grown farmers or volunteers, not a third-party inspector; mainly for farmers selling directly to consumers (farmer's markets), fewer fees, less paperwork

Global Animal Partnership:

- Started by Whole Foods and spreading to other stores
- Diet: Animals raised outdoors on pasture
- Living: No cages, crates, or tethers; living conditions have rigorous restrictions to ensure animals live in natural conditions
- Antibiotics/Hormones: No hormones, no antibiotics
- Other: They live on one farm their entire lives.

OTHER MEANINGLESS MARKETING LABELS YOU WILL SEE:

100% Natural:

- The FDA prohibits beef and lamb in this category to have any artificial colors, artificial flavors, preservatives, or other artificial ingredients. It does not specify or regulate how they are raised, what they eat, where they live or if they were given antibiotics.

Free-Range:

- This is only FDA regulated for chickens, but not for pigs, cattle, or egg producing chickens. There are different degrees of free-range, and they are not specified. It only means that the animal has access to the outdoors, but it does not mean that the animals have actually spent any time outdoors.

Raised Without Antibiotics:

- This is an unverified claim by third parties

American Humane Certified:

- Weakest of third-party verifications. [2]

Are There Benefits to Organic Meat?

- **Omega-3 fatty acids.** The feeding requirements for organic live-stock farming, such as the primary use of grass and alfalfa for cattle, result in generally higher levels of omega-3 fatty acids, a kind of fat that is more heart healthy than other fats. These higher omega-3 fatty acids are found in organic meats, dairy and eggs.

- **Bacteria.** Meats produced conventionally may have a higher occur-rence of bacteria resistant to antibiotic treatment. A 2015 study conducted by Consumer Reports compared 300 conventional and grass-fed meat samples. The findings: 18% of the conventionally grown meat was contaminated with antibiotic resistant bacteria as compared to 6% of grass-fed beef samples. [3,4,5,6,7]

- Many studies indicate that organic meats are safer and healthier than conventionally grown and processed meats. [16]

Medical Research on Antibiotics and Hormones in Animals.

- Of all the antibiotics sold in the US, 80% are used in the animal industry. Antibiotics used in raising animals are one of the main reasons for the antibiotic resistance seen in humans today.[8]

- 4 times more antibiotics are used in animals than humans.[9]

- Hormones and antibiotics help animals grow faster on diets that are poor and in conditions that are generally horrible.[10]

- Due to hormone exposure, cow udders get infected more often, thus requiring more antibiotics.[11]

- Due to subpar growing conditions, the animals get sick more often, necessitating antibiotic use.[12]

- Hormone and antibiotic use in animals are banned in all European nations, Australia, New Zealand, and Japan. [13,14,15]

MEAT SAMPLES TAINTED WITH INDICATOR BACTERIA

	TURKEY	PORK	BEEF	CHICKEN
Total samples tested	480	480	480	480
Number of samples contaminated with *Enterococcus faecalis*	392	334	269	186
Number of samples containing *Enterococcus faecalis* resistant to at least 1 antibiotic	389	332	263	185
Percent of meat samples containing antibiotic-resistant *Enterococcus faecalis*	**81%**	**69%**	**55%**	**39%**

Scientists study *Enterococcus* bacteria on meat to gauge fecal contamination and the spread of antibiotic-resistance traits.

Source: EWG calculations based on data drawn from the National Antimicrobial Resistance Monitoring System 2011 Retail Meat Report, published Feb. 5, 2013

Pro Tip:
Grass Fed Certified Meat by AWA Is the Best Choice

One More Thing, Let's Discuss Processed Meat:

The WHO and the International Agency for Research on Cancer (IARC) classify processed meat as IARC Group 1: Carcinogenic to humans.

- Note: Cigarette smoking is classified as Group 1 by the WHO. Does this mean that cigarettes and processed meats are equally carcinogenic? No. The IARC classification means that there is strong evidence to support the claim that processed meat and cigarette smoking cause cancer in humans.

- Processed meats refer to meat that has been transformed through salting, smoking, fermenting or processing the meat to enhance its flavor. The biggest culprits are nitrites.

- Processed meat examples: hot dogs (frankfurters), ham, sausages, corned beef, cold cuts, bacon, and biltong or beef jerky, as well as canned meat and meat-based preparations and sauces. Processed meats may contain red meats as well as poultry and fowl.

- Celery Powder and Celery products are naturally high in nitrates, so adding celery powder to meat is simply another way of providing nitrates. In passing from mouth to stomach, nitrates get converted to nitrites. So-called "nitrate-free" processed meats are often preserved with celery powder.

What does Harvard have to say on the matter of nitrates and nitrite free trend?

- The source of nitrate added for meat preservation will likely not matter. Furthermore, processed meats can contain other carcinogenic compounds such as PAHs which can be formed during smoking of meat (e.g. salami). Processed meats, particularly those containing red meat also contain heme iron, which can enhance the formation of carcinogenic compounds (NOCs) in the body. Until we know more about the exact mechanisms underlying the relationship between processed meat and cancers, it is best to treat those nitrate-free processed meats the same as any other processed meats and limit intake. [17]

How to Choose Affordable Grass Fed Organic Meat and Dairy:

- Organic meats, dairy, eggs, and produce can be found more and more at large wholesale warehouses such as Costco; organic produce can now be found at Walmart, Aldi, Target, etc.

- Thrive Market is an online discount grocery store.

- Sign up with your community for Azure Standard. It is an organization that delivers affordable organic food.

- Local farmers will sell entire parts of animals to families. You will need some good friends and a large freezer.

- Eat fewer animal products and more fruits and vegetables.

- Stop buying junk such as soda, Gatorade, juice, and Powerade and use the savings from these products to buy organic. Remember, water is nearly free and readily available.

- Buy in bulk and freeze what you don't need.

Eat red meat fewer than 5 times per month or about once a week.

For my mega list of shopping items from Costco, Walmart, Trader Joe's, Target, Aldi, etc. scan the code for my book resources page.

13

The Chicken or The Egg?

Unscrambling Egg and Chicken Labels

For years I pined for my own chicken coop which would produce fresh eggs daily. In fact, at one point I had my husband downloading "build your own chicken coop plans." After our neighbor attempted to raise chickens and explained to us the issues with coyotes, hawks, cats, the endless amount of chicken poop, the smell, and the fact you need a "chicken sitter" when you leave town, we decided maybe just making better egg choices at the store was the way to go.

How do you select eggs? Do you break into a sweat in the egg department? Here are some tips to help you understand what each label actually means.

Organic

- Label regulated by the USDA.

- Indicates that the food or other agricultural product has been produced through approved methods for cultural, biological, and mechanical practices.

- Synthetic fertilizers, sewage sludge, irradiation, and genetic engineering may not be used.

Outdoor access

- Label is meaningless.

- It does not mean the hens actually go outdoors.

- It can mean that there's a small door, which, if opened, would mean the hens could access the outdoors.

- There are actually no space requirements.

Non-GMO

- This only means that hens are fed a diet that is free from GMO's.

- That does not mean that the food is organic nor does it imply anything else.

Vegetarian Fed

- Hens aren't officially vegetarians. They eat insects such as worms and grubs.

- This essentially means that the feed they're given doesn't have animal byproducts, like ground up chicken.

Cage-free

- This label is regulated by the USDA.

- Hens can move freely within the building/hen house and have unlimited access to food and fresh water during their production cycle.

- There are no space requirements.

Certified Humane status

- There must be 1.5 square feet of space per hen, litter for dust bathing, perches for the birds, and ammonia levels at a maximum of 10 ppm which means the scent is imperceptible.

Free Range

- Misleading term
- Means that the hens must have access to the great outdoors for an indeterminate amount of time
- Not regulated
- It can simply imply that birds living indoors in overcrowded conditions had a tiny door that was open to the outdoors for a small amount of time

Pasture-raised

- This label is not regulated by the USDA.
- 108-square-feet per bird per Certified Humane Standards.
- Raised by Certified Humane Standards.

Natural

- This label means nothing.
- It claims to use no added hormones.
- Federal regulations have never allowed the use of hormones or steroids in poultry, pork, or goats.

Humane

- This is also not regulated by the USDA and doesn't mean much.

Animal Welfare Approved

- This focuses on smaller purveyors.
- Farmers can't have a flock of more than 500 birds.

My Favorite Eggs: (Non-sponsored)

https://www.peteandgerrys.com/organic-eggs/organic-egg

Cracking the Code on Poultry Labels.

The following are **useless** terms:

Natural

- It only implies that it is free of artificial color or ingredients
- It says nothing about how the chicken was raised or what it was fed

Hormone Free

- Useless labels since hormones are never allowed in poultry

Antibiotic-Free

- The farmer must produce documentation that no antibiotics were used to treat disease or as prophylaxis

Naturally Raised

- Means absolutely nothing. It does not indicate the living conditions or the feed quality for the chicken

Vegetarian Fed

- Useless term as well since chickens cannot be fed animal products. It might mean that the birds were not roaming free eating bugs and worms which is a natural part of their diet

Free-range

- This label is regulated by the USDA.

- Chickens must have continuous access to the outdoors during their production cycle, which may or may not be fenced and/or covered with a type of netting material.

- There is no stipulation as to what that outdoor access really means, or how much space is required.

The following are **helpful** terms:

Humanely Raised

- Term is regulated by the Humane Farm Animal Care Organization, not USDA

- Chickens are allowed to be, well, chickens. They can perch, peck, scratch, and forage for food

Pasture Raised

- Term regulated by the Humane Farm Animal Care Organization, not USDA

- Birds are raised outdoors year-round with access to shelter to be protected from inclement weather and predators

Organic

- Term regulated by the USDA

- Chickens must be fed a diet free of antibiotics, arsenic, hormones, animal by-products, synthetic fertilizers or pesticides

- It does not outline the living conditions

There are 5 egg labels you need to know and purchase if possible: organic, free range, certified humane, family farm, and animal welfare approved. There are 3 labels for poultry: organic, humanely raised, and pasture raised

For my mega list of shopping items from Costco, Walmart, Trader Joe's, Target, Aldi, etc. scan the code for my book resources page.

14

Need an Oil Change?

Cooking Oils: The Good, the Bad, and the Ugly

Our kids absolutely love fried chicken. Doesn't everyone? They used to get their fix at Chick-Fil-A until I realized how many chemicals are in their chicken. So, I began making my own with lots of vegetable oil, believing this was much healthier. For years I slowly changed the recipe opting for fewer processed ingredients. Fast forward many meals and now I use olive oil or avocado oil, organic chicken and home-made gluten free breadcrumbs. And they are still the biggest hit of my cooking repertoire!

We have all read and heard about the importance of fruits, vegetables, grains, and protein but where does fat come into play? For a while it seemed that low fat diets were all the rage and anything containing fat was to be avoided. It was assumed that eating fat created fat in the body, so people avoided it, substituting chemicals and all sorts of other substances to replace the fat in food. We now know that fat does not create fat and can actually help us lose weight. That said, a little oil can be part of a healthy diet.

Unfortunately, most of the processed foods we eat today are made from unhealthy hydrogenated and polyunsaturated oils. That's because these oils are much cheaper to make and help increase profitability for food companies. Therefore, before consuming oils it is important to know that not all oils are created equal and consuming certain oils can be downright dangerous to your health.

TYPES OF FATS:

Before we talk about which oils are good for you and which are not, it is important to have a basic understanding of fats. Fats can be broken down into 4 categories:

- Trans fats
- Polyunsaturated fats
- Monounsaturated fats
- Saturated fats

TRANS FATS:

- Labeled as hydrogenated and partially hydrogenated oil.
- Present in many processed foods and fast foods.
- Made by combining hydrogen with polyunsaturated oils.
- Dangerous and can cause a myriad of health problems.
- Increase the risk of heart disease drastically. These oils are in fact so dangerous that New York City banned the use of them in restaurants in 2007 and many cities are now doing the same.
- Still present in many processed foods.
- Can be present up to a half gram in food labeled trans fat-free.
- Present in any food containing partially hydrogenated oils.

POLYUNSATURATED FATS AND OILS:

- Probably the trickiest to understand.
- Essential to our bodies.
- Cannot be produced by the human body.
- Contain omega 3 and omega 6 fatty acids.
- Best to get these through whole foods and not oil.
- Examples we want to avoid include, vegetable oil, corn oil, canola

oil, safflower oil, soybean oil, sunflower oil

- The problem with polyunsaturated oils is that they form free radicals during the extraction process or when heated for cooking.

- Free radicals are known to initiate diseases such as cancer.

- The other major problem with these oils is that they contain an extremely uneven ratio of omega 6 to omega 3's.

- One of the major causes of inflammation in the US is due to the increase of omega 6 in our food consumption and lack of omega 3.

- These oils are all extremely high in omega 6 and low in omega 3.

- Omega 6 is not bad for you and is essential to the body. However, it needs to be balanced with omega 3 or it causes inflammation. Optimally, we should strive for a 2:1 ratio of omega 6 to omega 3 in our diet (the average American is consuming a 16:1 ratio of omega 6 to omega 3!).

But wait, there's more. Let's look at how canola oil is made. Here's an overly simplified version of the process. [1]

- **Step 1**: Find some "canola seeds." Oh wait, they don't exist. Canola oil is made from a hybrid version of the rapeseed, most likely genetically modified and heavily treated with pesticides.

- **Step 2**: Heat the rapeseeds at unnaturally high temperatures so that they oxidize and are rancid before you ever buy them.

- **Step 3**: Process with a petroleum solvent to extract the oils.

- **Step 4:** Heat some more and add some acid to remove any nasty wax solids that formed during the first processing.

- **Step 5:** Treat the oil with more chemicals to improve the color.

- **Step 6:** Deodorize the oil to mask the horrific smell from the chemical processing.

Of course, if you want to take your vegetable oils one step further, just hydrogenate it until it becomes a solid. Now you have margarine in all its trans-fatty wonder. And yes, the American Heart Association recommends vegetable oil and margarine for those suffering from heart disease. To say that I am baffled is an understatement.

MONO AND SATURATED FATS

Both **mono** and **saturated** fat can be healthy when consumed in moderation and include oils like:

- olive oil
- avocado oil
- coconut oil
- ghee

Consider cooking and sautéing with:

- broth
- wine
- water

Read Labels

- WARNING: this can be extremely frustrating! When I learned about how bad these oils were for me and started looking for them on food labels, I was shocked at how many of the foods I bought contained corn, safflower, sunflower, and soybean oil. Eliminating these oils can be very difficult if you purchase packaged foods and snacks. I recommend starting small and slowly cutting back on these oils by tackling one food product at a time, so you don't get overwhelmed.

How to Choose a Good Olive Oil [1]

- Look for a certified origin. For example, California Olive Oil

Commission (COOC), or the North American Olive Oil Association's (NAOOA), which bear a red circular logo with a green olive branch, International Olive Council (IOC).

- Purchase oils in dark-colored glass bottles. This helps reduce oxidation. Steer clear of plastic and light/clear bottles. Some international oils come in tins.

- Look for a harvesting date or pressing date on the label. This is not an expiration date. Try to get one within 6-12 months.

- Look for 100% extra virgin, 1st cold-pressed, and organic.

- Ideally, buy oil that's from a single origin or one source.

- **Beware** that olive oil heated over 320 degrees has the potential to degrade into carcinogenic compounds such as lipid peroxides and aldehydes.

- **Beware** of olive oils contaminated with cheaper refined olive oils.

- I use it in cooking, salad dressings, and roasting at lower temperatures.

How to Choose a Good Avocado Oil [2,3]

- It should taste grassy, buttery, and a little bit like mushrooms.

- Buy only those in tinted glass.

- Choose cold-pressed, steam-refined, or expeller-pressed.

- As a general rule, if an oil doesn't specify a higher-quality extraction method, it's usually a good indication that chemical or heat extraction was used.

- Virgin avocado oil should be green in color. Refined oil has pigments removed during refining; thus, it is light yellow and almost clear.

- Store in cool, dark cabinet, not next to the stove.

- Choose an oil that's closest to the harvest/production time to ensure maximum freshness. Use within 6 months.

- Beware some oils are diluted with soybean oil, high oleic sunflower or safflower oils.

- Beware that there are no industry standards.

- I use it for frying and roasting at high temperatures.

How to Choose Coconut Oil:

- Since it is a saturated fat, it is surrounded by controversy. Studies isolating coconut oil as the only saturated fat in a person's diet and its long-term effects, have not been done.

- It's a good source of MCT oil.

- Coconut oil is a good choice for high temperature cooking.

- If you want to use coconut oil at <u>high temperatures buy refined coconut oils.</u> Look for oils that have been refined using "chemical-free" methods or organic since the organic label prevents the use of harmful chemicals in the refining process

- <u>Unrefined oils</u> are best used for <u>lower temperature</u> cooking at less than 350 degrees Fahrenheit or for uncooked foods. Look for virgin, extra-virgin, or cold-pressed. You don't need to buy organic unrefined since this nut is not a source of high pesticide residue.

- I don't use this oil in my cooking because I don't like the taste.

What About Ghee?

- Ghee is a clarified type of butter. Its smoke point is on the higher side and is safe for cooking at 485 degrees Fahrenheit.

- It is a saturated fat.

- It is casein free. This makes it easier to digest for those with a dairy sensitivity

- I use it interchangeably with my dairy free alternatives, but not frequently since I have found many dairy free alternatives we love.

Avoid These Oils	
We shall term them "illegal"	
Canola Oil	Rapeseed Oil
Vegetable Oil	Sunflower Oil
Safflower Oil	Grapeseed Oil
Palm Oil	Soybean Oil
Corn Oil	Cottonseed Oil

Choose from These Olive Oils	
Kirkland Organic	Terra Delyssa Organic
Ellora Extra Virgin Olive Oil	Corto EVOO
California Olive Ranch	McEvoy Ranch Organic
Lucero	Partanna Extra Virgin Olive Oil
Cobram Estate	Lodi Frantoio Extra Virgin Olive Oil

Choose from These other Oils	
Coconut Oils	Avocado Oils
Nutiva Organic Virgin Coconut Oil	Avohass Avocado Oil
Viva Naturals Organic Extra-Virgin Coconut Oil	Marianne's Avocado Oil
Carrington Farms Organic Coconut Oil	Chosen Foods Avocado Oil
Anjou Coconut Oil	Nutiva Organic Avocado Oil
Nature's Way Coconut Oil	

Limit packaged foods containing "illegal oils" to fewer than 5 times a week.

For my mega list of shopping items from Costco, Walmart, Trader Joe's, Target, Aldi, etc. scan the code for my book resources page.

15

Arsenic for Dummies

Answers to All of Your Burning Questions About Arsenic

When I hear the word arsenic, I classically visualize the assassin carefully preparing his serum to complete the poisoning task. In fact, it was the poison of choice for murder in 19th century Britain! Thus, my children are always fascinated when I mention the presence of arsenic in rice or juice. Use this chapter to begin a novel dinner conversation with kids about the good and bad things which may be in our food.

Where Does Arsenic Come From?

- Arsenic is in pesticides applied to cotton and orchards since 1940.

- It comes in two chemical forms, organic and inorganic. The inorganic form of arsenic is cancer causing.

- Organic fields that no longer use pesticides and herbicides still have high levels of arsenic in the soil and water from previous pesticide/herbicide use.

- It has been put in chicken feed since 1940 as a growth promoter, color enhancer, and disease preventer. The arsenic is digested then is excreted in chicken waste which is consequently used as fertilizer and cattle feed. [1] In 2014, the FDA called for the removal of the animal drug Roxarsone from chicken feed because it can transform into inorganic arsenic. But progress is slow.

- It was present in pressure-treated wood used in residential housing. This was banned in 2003.

- Paints and dyes contain arsenic.

- Contaminated waste, herbicides, and pesticides leak into the soil which then leak into the water source, and this leads to contaminated drinking water, grains, and rice.

How Do We Know That Arsenic Is a Problem and Not Just a Social Media Rumor?

- In Chile and Bangladesh, arsenic contaminated water from deep wells was introduced into the city water supply to address the issue of chronic diarrheal disease. A large study in 2006 found that chronic exposure to arsenic in these populations led to skin changes, skin nodules, skin cancer, lung and bladder cancer, problems with neurological and behavioral development, chronic lung disease, such as bronchiectasis, and Type 2 diabetes. These findings were most obvious in fetuses and young children. [2]

- In 2006, a cross-sectional study showed a dose-dependent reduction in intellectual function in 10-year-olds. In other words, the higher the dose and the longer the exposure to arsenic, the lower the IQ, the lower the performance in school, and the greater the issues with behavior. [3]

How Do We Decrease Our Exposure to Arsenic in Water?

- Well water needs to be tested.

- In 2006, water standards were created for wells and city water. In most states, safe levels of inorganic arsenic in the water supply should be less than 10 parts per billion (ppb).

- Filter your water. For water filter options, please visit the chapter on Fluoride.

What's the Deal with Arsenic in Rice?

- Rice is a grain that is grown in water and tends to absorb arsenic very easily. It doesn't matter if it's organic or conventionally grown. All rice absorbs arsenic from the soil and water.

The following chart shows where many common grains fall in arsenic levels:

Low Arsenic Grains	
White rice	Farro
Sushi Rice from USA	Millet
Basmati Rice from California, India, Pakistan	Buckwheat
Quinoa	Polenta
Millet	Grits
Amaranth	Farley
Bulgur	
High Arsenic Grains	
Rice from Arkansas, Texas, Louisiana, Bangladesh	Brown Rice*

*Brown rice has 80% more arsenic than white rice, but more nutrients as well. Brown basmati from California, India, or Pakistan is the best choice with 1/3 less arsenic then other brown rice. [5,6]

Am I getting too much arsenic in my diet?

Product	Serving Size	Child Points	Adult Points
Infant Rice Cereal	1/4 cup, uncooked	1	NA
Rice Cereal, Hot	1/4 cup, uncooked	8	4
Rice Cereal, Ready to Eat	1 cup	5	2
Rice Drinks	1 cup	4	2
White Basmati or Sushi Rice	1/4 cup, uncooked	3	2
All Other Rice	1/4 cup, uncooked	6	4
Rice Pasta	2 ounces, uncooked	7	3
Rice Cakes	1 to 3 rice cakes	6	3
Rice Crackers	16 to 18 crackers	3	1
Cake or Muffin Mix	2 to 3 ounces	4	2
Brownie Mix	1 to 2 ounces	1	1
Cookies	1 to 3 cookies	2	1
Rice Pudding	about 1/3 cup	2	1
Pie- or Pizza-Crust Mix	2 ounces	2	1
Snack Bars (Cereal, Granola, or Energy)	1- to 2-ounce bar	3	1

*Table is based on the article published in the January 2015 Consumer Reports, though point values have been rounded. [4][7]

MY RULE: FEWER THAN 5 POINTS PER WEEK.

Thanks for the Scientific Data, but We're Still Confused. What Do We Do to Be Safe?

- No rice cereal for babies. None.

- Fruits and veggies should be the first foods for babies. From scratch. Examples are avocados, bananas, sweet potatoes. Whatever you're eating that can be mashed up. Don't make it too complicated.

- Use oatmeal cereal as a thickener for baby foods if needed.

- Avoid baby formulas, toddler formulas, and toddler snacks with brown rice syrup.

- Do not use rice milk as an alternative to dairy. Unsweetened almond milk is a great alternative.

- Read labels and avoid rice syrup sweeteners.

- Beware that gluten free products have various processed rice additives such as rice flour, rice syrup, etc.

- Use a variety of grains such as quinoa, bulgur, and millet as suggested above.

- Review the chart above as a guide for rice consumption.

Should You Change the Way You Cook Rice?

- Traditionally, people rinse rice then cook it in sufficient water that is absorbed during simmering. Rinsing rice before cooking has a minimal effect on the arsenic content of the cooked grain but it removes most of the nutrients in rice. However, cooking rice in extra water then draining like pasta, reduces average inorganic arsenic by 40% from long grain polished, 60% from parboiled and 50% from brown rice. [8,9]

Where Else Is Arsenic a Problem?

- Due to the pesticides and herbicides used in orchards and vineyards, apple and grape juices have high levels of arsenic. The fruits themselves contain low levels of this chemical. [10] However, when fruits get juiced and boiled together, especially fruits imported from other countries, it leads to concentrated levels of arsenic.[11]

- A majority of children drink two to five times this recommended amount. Unless you juice at home, I recommend none. Urine studies in children who drink juice daily show levels of arsenic above the 10 ppm, the recommended safe threshold in drinking water. [12]. The FDA approved 10 ppm as the safe threshold of arsenic in apple juice. [13]

Once Again Great Info, but What Do We Do?

- Stop buying apple and grape juice.

- Make juice at home from locally grown and organic apples and grapes.

- Don't allow daily juice in daycares and preschools. Speak with the schools. NYC has already passed a law prohibiting this. If enough parents speak up, the daycares will stop. Juice is cheap, milk is not. But hey, water is free!

- Do not give juice to babies and toddlers.

- Water and milk are best! An occasional juice here and there is no big deal but keep it to four to six ounces max per day. Can we just stop with the overuse of juice already?!?

- No juice boxes in kids' lunches.

- Avoid foods with rice syrup.

- Apples have tremendous health impacts and should be part of the daily diet. Grapes have amazing health benefits and should be eaten regularly. Eat the fruit, not the store-bought juice.

I recommend children consume rice and products containing rice fewer than 5 times per week.

For my mega list of shopping items from Costco, Walmart, Trader Joe's, Target, Aldi, etc. scan the code.

16

You Lyte Up My Life

Electrolytes and Sports Drinks

Have you ever wondered why children need an entire meal at halftime of their kiddie sports events with copious amounts of uber-hydrating sports drinks to treat their presumed severe dehydration? If your kids are anything like mine, they sat in the backfield picking grass and singing most of the time. Why is finishing the game rewarded with a giant box of donuts or cupcakes? I remember one of my kid's teammates telling him that it doesn't matter if we win or lose, just what the snack is at the end of the game! I contacted our local youth sport's organization in an attempt to change the practice of the "snack parent" and the sugar laden sports drinks and I was quickly labelled a problem parent by the organization. Interestingly, during our time in New Zealand, water seemed to work just fine to get our kids through the games!

A LESSON ON GATORADE

In 1965, University of Florida (UF) football coach Dwayne Douglas noticed that his players were losing a lot of weight during training and games, some up to 18 pounds (8.1 kilograms)! They weren't urinating despite drinking a lot of water and players were suffering from heat stroke. Douglas teamed up with Dr. Robert Cade, a kidney disease specialist at UF, to talk the problem out. Cade worked with UF's College of Medicine to develop a drink to replenish what these athletes were losing through their sweat: carbohydrates (A.K.A. sugar), salt and electrolytes. Electrolytes are a set of minerals that your body needs to maintain healthy fluid levels and regulate its muscle function.[1] The only problem was that the drink tasted disgusting, so Cade's wife proposed adding lemon juice to make it a little more palatable. This was all well and good until Quaker Oats got involved in 1983, then Pepsi bought Quaker Oats in 2001. What started out as a great solution to a serious problem became a marketing phenomenon plagued by chemicals and greed. Needless to say, I **never** recommend Gatorade.

Original Gatorade Ingredients	
First Batch	Second Batch Added These for Taste
Water	Cyclamate (sweetener)
Sodium Citrate (salt)	Lemon
Monopotassium	
Fructose (sugar)	

Current Gatorade Formula	
Water	Citric Acid
Sodium Citrate	Gum Arabic
Monopotassium Phosphate	Glycerol Ester of Rosin
Sugar	Natural Flavor
Dextrose	Yellow 5

The Electrolyte Story

Why Do We Need Electrolytes?

- Our cells need fluids and electrolytes to function properly.
- Electrolytes are electrically charged minerals and compounds that help our muscles, nerves, and organs function properly.

- Examples of electrolytes are potassium (K+), sodium (Na+), magnesium (Mg+), etc.

Who Needs Electrolytes?

- Everyone needs electrolytes.

- Electrolytes, along with hydration, are important to have all the time but especially when children are active, have diarrhea, or are spending time in hot environments.

But Should You Indulge in Gatorade the Way Commercials Encourage You To?

- Look at how electrolytes compare in Gatorade vs. Food in the graph below.

- The marketing world has made us believe that nothing out there compares to Gatorade when it comes to rehydration for the stomach bug or after a tough practice on the sports field.

- They even convinced us that the only way to become remotely athletic is to drink Gatorade.

- I am confused as to why a sick child needs artificial food coloring. More on food coloring in a later chapter.

- As a refresher on sugar: The human body can only process 24 grams of added sugar per day. Fruits have natural sugar and sports drinks have added sugar.

- Here are how sports drinks compare to real food:

Electrolytes	Powerade	Gatorade	Grapes	Orange	Apple	Banana	Coconut water*
Potassium	60mg	75mg	294mg	250mg	179mg	422mg	514gm
Sodium	250mg	270mg	2.5mg	1mg	1mg	1.2mg	4mg
Added Sugar (Bad)	34gm	34gm					
Natural Sugar (Good)			24gm	13gm	19gm	14gm	12gm
Protein	0	0	1.1gm	1.4gm	0.5gm	1.3gm	0
Carbohydrate	35gm	34gm	25gm	18gm	24gm	27gm	14gm
Fiber	0	0	2.9gm	3.9gm	3.4gm	3gm	1gm

*Harmless Harvest Brand

HOMEMADE GATORADE RECIPE

Ingredients:

- 32 oz of green tea, herbal tea, Harmless Harvest Coconut Water or plain water
- 1/4 tsp Himalayan salt
- 1 tsp unflavored Natural Calm Calcium-Magnesium Powder
- 1/4 cup 100% raw, unpasteurized juice or 1-2 Tbsp raw honey

Instructions:

- Steep the tea or warm water/coconut water slightly.
- Mix all ingredients except the honey. Adjust honey to taste.
- Be careful, flavored Natural Calm is sweetened with stevia and other flavors. If you choose to use this, make sure you taste the concoction before you add honey.

Electrolyte Breakdown of Ingredients:

- 32 oz of Harmless Harvest Organic Coconut Water

- 45mg sugar
- 120mg calcium
- 1620mg potassium
- 1/4 tsp Himalayan salt
- 575mg sodium
- 1 tsp Natural Calm Calcium-Magnesium Powder
- 85mg vitamin C
- 35 IU vitamin D3
- 70mg calcium
- 103mg magnesium
- 32mg potassium
- 88mg boron
- 1 Tbsp honey
- 16 grams sugar

Drink only homemade sports drinks with fewer than 5 ingredients.

For my mega list of shopping items from Costco, Walmart, Trader Joe's, Target, Aldi, etc. scan the code

17

Keeping it Real

How Food Companies Hijack Our Taste Buds

A long time ago, I was under the illusion that my kids were eating healthy. They had a warm breakfast such as toaster strudel (with their names creatively written in icing). Their lunch was "well balanced" with a Smucker's Uncrustibles sandwich (protein), apple sauce (fruit), Danimals yogurt drink (calcium), and Cheetos (a crunch like the other kids so they didn't feel different). Snacks were a legit fruit and Jello (the jiggly food group) or Kozy Shack rice pudding (protein). Dinner was "homemade" and by that, I mean that I opened a bag of Bertolli frozen dinner and cooked it on the stove. This chemical concoction did not seem absurd because I was reading only the front of packages and believed their marketing. Once I learned to read the back of containers and to scour the ingredient list, I became horrified at what I was feeding my family. I had facilitated a massive chemical craving in my family! As a response I tried a dramatic food shift but was met with a swift and emphatic rebellion. I changed course and began to substitute one whole food at a time. It was slow, painful at times, but in the end successful.

By now you realize that choosing food is confusing and understanding the chemical smorgasbord added to many of our processed food items is overwhelming. Remember, these food additives are made in a lab by a scientist. The goal is to make these substances so incredible that there is always a party in our mouths, and we are left ready to purchase the next bag or cookie. Mother nature simply makes a potato. She is not in the business of making money. Furthermore, taste buds are supposed to protect us from danger, such as poisonous berries or mushrooms. All this mucking around with food chemicals has confused our taste buds into thinking that chemicals are safe and good for us to eat. I know, I know, there are a lot of naysayers on this one. I often hear, "I used to eat the same foods when I was little and I'm fine. What's the big deal? "

Unfortunately, this could not be farther from the truth. The food we ate 30 years ago is not the same food we are eating today. Over 10,000 food preservatives have been added to our food since the 1980's. Even scarier, most of these have not been tested on humans. They have been grandfathered in under the Generally Recognized as Safe (GRAS) designation without FDA approval or notification. The Academy of Pediatrics urges doctors and parents to be aware of the lack of data on children's hormones, neurological, and biological development, and these food additives. [1]

Here is a great example:

Kellogg's Frosted Flakes before 1996

- Corn and sugar

Regular Frosted Flakes 2020:

- GMO corn, GMO sugar, BHT for freshness, salt, malt flavor, iron, niacinamide, palmitate, folic acid, vitamin D, vitamin B12, riboflavin, pyridoxine hydrochloride, ascorbic acid, sodium ascorbate

Organic Frosted Flakes 2020:

- Organic milled corn, organic cane sugar, sea salt

To make your life easier, I am going to outline several food ingredients that you need to avoid. I will keep it simple and straightforward. You will find the detailed research in the reference section. My goal is to simplify your understanding. At the end of the list, you will find a handy-dandy way to make your life and shopping easier.

Artificial Flavors and Natural Flavors

- Artificial flavors appear on one out of every seven food labels and natural flavors appears on over 80,000 food labels. Artificial flavors are a chemical experiment that should be avoided. Natural flavors are trickier because they can contain synthetic chemicals such as the solvent propylene glycol or the preservative BHA. But wait, the food company does not have to tell us where the natural flavor comes from if it is from a plant or an animal. My favorite example is the natural flavor, Castoreum, a substance that comes from a gland near a beaver's butt. This is used as a vanilla, strawberry, or raspberry flavor in ice cream, chewing gum, pudding and brownies. [2]

Artificial Colors

- Blue 2, green 3, red 3, red 40, yellow 5, and yellow 6 are found in many foods like cereals, gum, candy, pickles, condiments and even children's liquid medications, toothpaste, and adult pills. Artificial colors have been shown to cause hyperactivity and inattention in groups of children who are susceptible. These dyes are banned in Norway and Austria and contain warnings in the UK and The European Union. [3]

Caramel Coloring

- The most widely used food coloring in the world. It's found in beer, soda, yogurts, cereal, granola bars, etc. The concern is that the compound 4-methylimidazole (4-MEI) is formed during the manufacturing of some caramel colors and is a carcinogen. [4]

Potassium Bromate

- Ingredient found in crackers and bread. It helps dough rise. It is deemed a carcinogen and a probable carcinogen by the state of California and by the International Cancer Agency. This ingredient is banned by the UK, Canada, and The European Union. However, in the US, we still allow it to be added to flour. [5]

Nitrites and Nitrates

- Ingredients which are used in food to retain color, or as preservatives and flavor enhancers. Have you ever wondered how salami stays pink for weeks and weeks on shelves? These are found in cured meats such as bacon, salami, sausages and hot dogs. Nitrites are deemed a probable carcinogen by the WHO. [6]

Propylparaben

- Used to extend shelf life without germ contamination in foods such as tortillas, muffins and food dyes. In 2010, a federal study found that 91% of Americans tested positive for this chemical in their urine. This chemical acts like a weak estrogen, causing issues with fertility in women, decreased sperm count, decreased testosterone, and it has been reported to speed up the growth of breast cancer cells. [7]

Butylated Hydroxyanisole (BHA)

- Found in packaging materials, cereals, sausage, hot dogs, meat patties, chewing gum, potato chips, beer, butter, vegetable oils, cosmetics and animal feed. It preserves the color of "food" and extends its shelf life. Unfortunately, the state of California has deemed it a carcinogen and the WHO considers it a potential carcinogen. Studies done in animals show it to lower testosterone and the thyroid hormone, thyroxine, decrease the quality of sperm, and cause behavioral issues. These are banned in Australia, New Zealand, Japan, Europe. [8]

Butylated Hydroxytoluene (BHT)

- The cousin of BHA. It is used to extend shelf life of foods just like BHA. It has been shown to increase tumor growth in several animal studies, increase behavioral issues in offspring, and affect testosterone and thyroid function. It is especially toxic when combined with BHA in food. Lastly, this is also banned from Australia, New Zealand, Japan, Europe. [9]

T-Butylhydroquinone (TBHQ)

- Extends the shelf life of foods by maintaining color and preventing rancidity. It is found in crackers and cereal. Though the FDA considers this a safe ingredient, TBHQ has been linked to food allergies such as nuts, milk, eggs, wheat and shellfish. [10]

Propyl Gallate

- Used as a preservative in products that contain animal fats, such as sausage and lard, and in vegetable oils. Some data suggests it may have weak estrogen activity, thus interfering with sex hormones. Animal data shows this chemical to increase cancer. [11,12]

Theobromine

- Found in cocoa, chocolate beverages and in chocolate-based foods such as cereal. The data shows developmental and reproductive issues, such as testicular atrophy in animals. [13]

The Takeaway:

Okay, okay, you are probably overwhelmed right now. Fear not, I've got your back. Better yet, the EWG does. They have created a food rating system called "Food Scores" and "less than 5 is your answer."

https://apps.apple.com/us/app/ewgs-food-scores/id930172079

A quick tutorial before you get to the QR code:

- Go to the page: https://www.ewg.org/foodscores/ or scan QR

- Enter the food of choice in the search bar.

- A category list will pop up. Pick the category, and another list will pop up based on concerns about nutrition, ingredients, and processing.

- The scale is 1-10 with 1 being the cleanest and 10 being the worst.

Any food you eat should have an EWG score lower than 5.

For my mega list of shopping items from Costco, Walmart, Trader Joe's, Target, Aldi, etc. scan the code for my book resources page.

18

Don't Let Your Sweet Emotion Get the Best of You

Understanding Sugar and Its Substitutes

I would have never guessed that changing our peanut butter would be construed as such an underhanded move by my family. Living in Romania, peanut butter was non-existent, so I really had a poor understanding of the importance of peanut butter in the American lifestyle. My husband was raised on PB & J and considers himself something of a peanut butter aficionado. When I looked at the amount of sugar added to the typical American peanut butter I was appalled. So, I made the logical choice to buy natural organic peanut butter, unaware that it pours out of the jar like oil. The first lunch of PB & J sandwiches made with my liquid peanut butter turned the dining table into a Pearl Harbor-like scene. John once again accused me of "removing all the joy from my life". This led to a whole series of family peanut butter blind taste-testings, sandwich trials, and even a black-market closet of illegal peanut butters. But as usual, my persistence led us to find the Goldilocks of peanut butters, consistency without the sugar!

The human body can only process a certain amount of sugar per day:

- 9 packets or 36 grams per day for men

- 6 packets or 24 grams per day for women and children [1]

Some Sugar Facts

- Sugar is everywhere and it's an uphill battle
- Sugar is very addictive
- Sugar is unfortunately closely associated with the happiness of childhood

Remember that there is natural sugar in various forms from our foods - fruits, dairy, veggies, grains. However, natural sugar from these items is metabolized differently than sugar from table sugar, agave, corn syrup, and honey.

Why is sugar an issue?

- Many of you have already heard me discuss how just 100gms of sugar decreases immune system function for up to 5hrs after ingestion. 100gms = 2 slices of cake, can of soda, or 10oz of OJ (think Birthday party).
- You know that sugar puts us at risk for diabetes, obesity, heart disease, but what about the brain.
- What you might not know is that added sugar in a child's diet is associated with sleep disruption, behavior issues, memory, impulsivity, and anxiety.

Did you know that sugar shrinks the brain?

- First, our brain and body need sugar to function. The brain, in fact, uses about ½ of the sugar energy from the body. But too much of a good thing is irritating to this delicate organ
- The most profound effects of sugar on the brain are found in people with diabetes and pre-diabetes. That does not mean those folks are the only ones affected. It does not mean, let's wait until we have diabetes and if we don't have diabetes our brains are fine. Not so fast ....

- A study in 103 children ages 7–11 years old showed that increased sugar intake was associated with alterations in hippocampal structure and connectivity in children based on MRI imaging. [1] What?????

- Too much sugar can interfere with how neurons, brain cells, talk to each other, nerve signal transmission, nerve cell activity and brain wave functions

- Too much sugar has been shown to interfere with memory and cognition in rats and adults, and lead to smaller brains, even in those without diabetes

THE HIPPOCAMPUS is very sensitive to sugar overload

- Many rat and adult studies have confirmed that a diet high in sugar leads to abnormal brain function. [2][2a]

- Hundreds of studies in rats have also shown brain shrinkage from too much sugar in the diet[3]

- One study showed that people who eat a western diet, but do not have diabetes, have a smaller hippocampus then those who consumed a healthy diet - fresh vegetables, salad, fruit, and grilled fish [4]

Effects of Sugar on the brain include:

- Impacts Memory, (ADD) [5]

- Effects on Mood, (tantrums)

- Hinders Mental Capacity (Learning issues) [6]

- Reduces the production brain-derived neurotrophic factor (BDNF), a brain chemical essential for new memory formation and learning [7]

What can you do?

- No ADDED sugar for kids less than 2 years old

- Baby and Toddler brains are very susceptible to negative effects from sugar

No candy in the classroom

- Parents please provide stickers, erasers, figurines, or coins for teachers to give as rewards

- If candy is in the classroom, have your child bring home candy in exchange for small inexpensive gifts. Ex: for every 5 pieces of candy, she will get a sticker or a random trinket

- For Birthday parties consider other treats for the kids instead of doughnuts/cupcakes. Kids just want goodies and to be singled out for their birthday, it's not really about the cupcake. If you must have cupcakes, bring the bite size ones.

Starting in 2020, the FDA began implementing new food and beverage labels to state how much added sugar products contain.

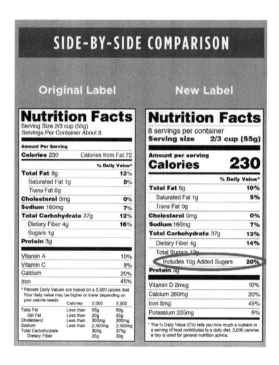

Here is a list of 56 alternate names for sugar found in "healthy" and "organic" foods that can fool you. There are 200 more names

not listed here:

The Many Names of Sugar			
Dextrose	Fructose	Galactose	Glucose
Lactose	Maltose	Sucrose	Beet sugar
Brown sugar	Cane juice crystals	Cane sugar	Castor sugar
Coconut sugar	Confectioner's sugar (aka powdered sugar)	Corn syrup solids	Crystalline fructose
Date sugar	Demerara sugar	Dextrin	Diastatic malt
Ethyl maltol	Florida crystals	Golden sugar	Glucose syrup solids
Grape sugar	Icing sugar	Maltodextrin	Muscovado sugar
Panela sugar	Raw sugar	Sugar (granulated or table)	Sucanat
Turbinado sugar	Yellow sugar	Agave Nectar/ Syrup	Barley malt
Blackstrap molasses	Brown rice syrup	Buttered sugar/ buttercream	Caramel
Carob syrup	Corn syrup	Evaporated cane juice	Fruit juice
Fruit juice & Fruit Juice concentrate	Golden syrup	High-Fructose Corn Syrup (HFCS)	Honey
Invert sugar	Malt syrup	Maple syrup	Molasses
Rice syrup	Refiner's syrup	Sorghum syrup	Treacle

Alternatives to Sugar Explained

The following are not considered added sugar

Pureed Fruits

- Contain fiber, vitamins, minerals, and natural sweetness

Dates, Date Sugar, Date Syrup

- These come from date palm trees and contain fiber, potassium, copper, iron, manganese, magnesium, and vitamin B6.

The following are better than table sugar and corn syrup, but they are still considered ADDED SUGAR.

Raw Dark Local Honey

- Full of enzymes, antioxidants, iron, zinc, potassium, calcium, phosphorus, vitamin B6, riboflavin and niacin
- Contains powerful antioxidants
- The darker the honey, the more nutrient dense it is
- Local honey provides you with oral tolerance to local pollen. In other words, it can help reduce reactions to pollen.
- Pasteurized honey loses some of its health benefits.

Maple Syrup

- Organic, pure maple syrup is full of antioxidants, manganese, riboflavin, zinc, magnesium, calcium, and potassium.
- Darker syrups contain more antioxidants than lighter syrups.

Coconut Sugar

- Extracted from the sap of the coconut flower, it is rich in polyphenols, iron, zinc, calcium, potassium, antioxidants, phosphorous and other phytonutrients.

Organic Blackstrap Molasses

- Highly nutritious, a great source of iron and calcium.

- Also rich in copper, potassium, manganese, selenium and vitamin B6.

- It comes from a third boiling of sugar cane which concentrates its nutrients.

THE STEVIA AND MONK DEBATE

Stevia Leaf Extract

- This plant is native to South America and is 200 times sweeter than sugar.

- It has become a marketing hot topic and there are many garbage versions of this product out there.

- Make sure there are no additives or preservatives present.

- Avoid liquid versions containing alcohol.

- Whether you choose powder or liquid make sure it consists of only one ingredient.

- Some stevia products have a bitter aftertaste and thus some stevia containing products may have other sweeteners added to counteract this like erythritol

- Stevia is not absorbed by the body, it travels all the way to the colon

- There is no glucose, and insulin isn't produced

Stevia Good News

- It does not directly cause weight gain or insulin spike

- Not carcinogenic

- Better then aspartame, sucralose, and other fake sugars

Stevia Bad News

Several studies show that Stevia adversely affects the gut microbiome [9][10]. It:

- Reduces the ammonium level

- Reduces the fermentative processes

- Increases the colonic pH

- This leads to fewer short-chain fatty acids (SCFAs)

- SCFA's are the main energy source of colon cells, making them crucial to gastrointestinal health

- SCFAs might influence gut-brain communication and brain function directly or indirectly [11]

- The most recent 2020 the study shows that stevia disrupts communications between different bacteria in the gut microbiome. It did not kill off the bacteria. Studies were done on stevia extract [12]

- The actual leaf of stevia is ok to use

Monk Fruit

- A small gourd which looks like a melon and is grown in Southeast Asia.

- It was originally used by monks in the 13th century, hence its name.

- It comes in various forms.

- Dextrose and erythritol (artificial sugar alcohols) are often added to monk fruit products which defeats the purpose of the natural product.

- These additional ingredients can cause stomach upset, vomiting and diarrhea

- Choose products with only one ingredient.

- Though it has zero calories, a low glycemic index, and has antioxidant properties, there is insufficient data to conclude its safety in humans [13]

- existing studies have not tested the specific effects of monk fruit on gut microbes

More Stevia and Monk Fruit Bad News

As mentioned, stevia and monk fruit are 150-300 times sweeter than sugar. Even when used in small doses, the effect on taste buds is powerful. The more stevia in the diet, the more we train our kid's taste buds to crave sugar, which leads to more sugary snacks, more white carbs, and more processed foods. And the whining continues, and the addiction worsens.

Also, many of us see Stevia and Monk fruit as "safe" or "not as bad as" sugar, giving us a sense of security, and allowing it to infiltrate our foods, lives, and bodies.

Moral of the story:

- Stevia and Monk fruit are sweeteners.
- They do not raise insulin levels
- They are to be counted as added sugar
- Evaluate your pantry and see how many "healthy" items have stevia or monk fruit
- In my house I do not use stevia, monk fruit, erythritol, allulose, etc. I use dates, sugar, honey, maple syrup with a goal to keep it under 24gms of added sugar per day

Examples of foods with hidden sugars:

- Pasta Sauce
- Energy Drinks
- Granola Bars

- BBQ Potato Chips
- Yogurt
- Salad Dressing
- Condiments
- Items with "kids" on the label
- "Sugar Free", "Zero Sugar" on the label

Eat fewer than 5 items with added sugar per day.

For my mega list of shopping items from Costco, Walmart, Trader Joe's, Target, Aldi, etc. scan the code for my book resources page.

19

Pour Some Sugar on Me

Why Store-Bought Juice is Sugar in Disguise

Juice boxes were a staple in my kids' lunchboxes. They were easy, cute, and kids loved them. Juice was one of the five main food groups which included: Lunchables as the protein, juice as the hydration, grapes as the fruit, Gogurt as the calcium and granola bars for crunch. One day, I added up the sugar content of my kid's lunchboxes and it totaled the amount they should have been allowed to consume in one week. I suddenly became aware that I was dousing them with tons of sugar in one meal, a meal at school, where they had to sit still and focus. At the same time, I was puzzled as to why my middle one was always in trouble with the teachers. Once I realized what my children were really eating, I started operation "Juice weaning." I started with doing juice boxes every other day. Then it was only on Tuesday/Thursdays. Then once a week. Then gone. There is nothing wrong with making changes slowly.

Most of us are fooled by juice companies. It's hard not to fall for the shiny labels and health claims such as:

- One to two servings of fruits and veggies per serving
- No added sugar
- 100% real juice
- Organic

Sounds healthy right? Sold? Not so fast. Here is the rest of the story on store-bought juice:

- Fruits and veggies are squeezed into a giant vat removing all fiber.
- The juice in vats is heated at high temperatures to kill bacteria per FDA regulations. This is called pasteurization.
- Once anything is boiled for a period of time, it loses its vitamins, minerals, and antioxidants.
- What remains is sugar.

The clever advertising by the juice companies results in people thinking they are choosing a nutritious beverage when in reality:

- Kids in day care are being served sugar in a sippy cup.
- Kids' lunch boxes contain sugar with a straw.
- Teens drink cans of sugar disguised as fruits and/or veggies.
- Parents provide their children with liquid sugar, believing it to be fruits and veggies.

Possible Counterarguments:

MyPlate.gov states that a glass of juice is considered a serving of fruit or veggies.

- It does not specify homemade juice.
- I would also like to add that the US Government considers pizza sauce to be a serving of vegetables. I rest my case!

But there will be so much whining in the house.

- Stop buying juice and the whining goes away in two or three days.
- If it's not in the house, kids will lose interest in futile whining.
- If you hide it, they will find it so good luck with that one!

But the kids get calcium and vitamin D from the OJ.

- Squeeze oranges and give them a drop of vitamin D (no taste, no smell, no color, no sugar).

- There is no need for a side of 12 packets of sugar with their vitamins.

It is okay to:

- Buy raw, unpasteurized juice.
- Make homemade juice; this is fabulous!!!
- Read the ingredient labels on all foods.
- Slowly dilute the juice over time until the result is a splash of juice in water. (See the juice dilution method discussed in the taste bud chapter)
- Infuse your water with fruits and herbs.
- Drink coconut water and kombucha
- Buy a juicer.

It is NOT okay to:

- Believe the claims on the fronts of boxes or bottles.
- Buy Roaring Waters thinking its water. This is sugar and water in a box; again, fabulous advertising.
- Buy juice because it has an organic label. This is organic sugar in a box. It still has to be pasteurized meaning it's been boiled to death.
- Buy juices because they claim to have less sugar (My guess is that they dilute the sugar in these products).

If you must buy juice, aim for fewer than 5 servings of juice per week.
1 serving = 5 ounces.

For my mega list of shopping items from Costco, Walmart, Trader Joe's, Target, Aldi, etc. scan the code for my book resources page.

20
Sugar Monsters
Dealing with the Halloween Candy Extravaganza

As far as I know we are the only country that pushes our kids to disguise themselves and go beg for candy from friends and neighbors with the goal of bagging as much loot as possible. To give our kids a competitive edge we sent them out with pillowcases rather than pumpkin buckets to maximize the ergonomics of collecting sweets. Given our initial policy of maximal candy collection, it's not surprising that I faced a full mutiny when I announced the 5-day limit on all candy stockpiled. My youngest child's solution was to keep an auxiliary candy bag which he then took to school and where he set up a black-market candy distribution system. While I was delighted with his entrepreneurial spirit, I was mortified that the health doctor's son was the ringleader of this middle school sugar empire. Humbling days.

Halloween is one of the most highly anticipated holidays for kids but at the end of the night, we are left with mountains of candy. Kids are obsessed. Parents are stressed. Some are delighted by the treats; others are horrified by the pounds of sugar brought into their homes. How do we keep the kids from devouring endless packages of KitKats and Reese's Peanut Butter Cups? How do we balance the sugar explosion with parental common sense? We can't just throw it away because that means we are disposing of happiness, money, deliciousness, a kid's right to indulge, and their hard-earned loot. Maybe we should look at this bounty as garbage, chemicals, food coloring, and loads of sugar.

10 Real-Life Ways to Tame the Candy Monsters We Create Each Halloween

1. Don't let kids leave the house without breakfast.

- Make sure kids have a breakfast containing proteins like eggs, uncured bacon, nitrite-free sausage, whole fat Greek yogurt, or peanut butter.

- Add fruit and whole-grain toast to complete the meal. Sugar cereal is not a good option.

2. Keep lunch simple.

- Pack a whole wheat sandwich with nitrite-free turkey or salami, cheese, lettuce, fruits or veggies on the side.

- A thermos of soup and a side of grapes.

- A nitrite-free turkey roll-up with cheese and red peppers.

- A candy treat this week will be okay. A "fun size" candy bar added to a simple, yet complete lunch will lead to less of a sugar rush. The sugar in the candy will be balanced by the fiber, protein, and fat in the lunch and will lead to less of a sugar spike, and less insulin means better digestion.

- *Don't* add juice, granola bars, chips, fruit gummies, fruit roll-ups, or crackers to the lunch as extras. These extras are added sugar that shouldn't be in a healthy lunch anyway, especially if Halloween candy is included. If the healthy part of the lunch is brought back home, then no candy should be sent the next day. The week of Halloween is a great opportunity to demonstrate to kids how we balance healthy eating with junk food.

3. Don't pack candy for snack time at school.

- Candy at snack time leads to a sugar rush, followed by a sugar crash. This results in a bad mood, talking out of turn, not focusing, acting like a clown, not finishing schoolwork, not paying attention, and a very unhappy and frustrated teacher.

Better snack ideas:

- Fruit or veggie family: dried apple slices, grapes, frozen blueberries
- Protein family: cheese sticks, nuts if allowed at school
- Complex carbohydrate family: whole wheat crackers or popcorn
- Goldfish crackers do not count because they lack fiber and simply turn to sugar after being eaten.
- See snack section for more ideas.

4. At the risk of sounding redundant, have fruits and veggies on the counter when kids get home from school.

- Their starving little selves will fill up on natural sugar from fruit before asking for the junk. Generally, they will eat what they see first. Kids are blinded to cut up fruit sitting in the fridge.

You can also keep a high protein snack on the counter such as:

- Pistachios
- Almonds
- Walnuts
- Steamed edamame or roasted, shelled edamame
- Guacamole
- Cheese
- Whole wheat cakes
- Whole fat Greek yogurt
- Rolled up nitrite-free cold cuts
- Apple slices with nut butter

** Go to Chapter 12, "Where is the Beef?" for more information

- These will fill them up on long-lasting nutrition and curb their need for those Reese's Pieces. If they are dying for a piece of candy, no big deal. They won't have room in their bellies for very much candy *and* the sugar from the candy will be balanced with fiber, protein, and fat for better absorption with less of a sugar rush. I am not a proponent of candy for snack. Just trying to be real.

5. Set expectations for how long candy is allowed in the house.

- My rule: 5 Days

- I am tempted by the candy, they are tempted, so we compromised. This does not mean bingeing daily for one week. We treat our bodies with respect. We feed our bodies with good nutrition but we will allow ourselves to indulge in the coveted candy for one week. There is no need to keep candy in the house for any longer than this set period. It just sets the stage for whining and complaining, not to mention the sugar rush side effects.

- During cold and flu season, the effects of sugar are much worse. To review: the more sugar we feed our bodies, the less immune response we will have to all those viruses and bacteria present in schools. This means more colds, sore throats, night-time coughs, congestion, and headaches, just to name a few symptoms associated with a sugar overload.

6. If you allow candy after dinner, set expectations for the amount of candy permitted.

- No whining, no bargaining, and no fuss. If they complain about your rule, they don't receive candy. Make sure that they eat a meal with protein, veggies, and complex carbs. Mac and cheese and frozen chicken nuggets are not a good meal choice. They need chicken, fish, beans, pork, etc. The proper serving size is one tablespoon per year of age for each food group: proteins, veggies, and complex carbs. No dinner means no candy. This is another great opportunity to discuss how we eat for health, not for fun.

156

7. Keep kids active after school.

- No sitting around watching TV, playing video games, and thinking about candy. Make sure they play outside and have plenty to do to keep them burning off the Halloween sugar overload.

- Playdates are a great way to keep them distracted. Going to a park after homework is done can also do the trick.

- Set up a scavenger hunt, such as: find 10 yellow leaves, 10 green leaves, 10 red leaves, 20 acorns, 5 sticks, 7 rocks, etc.

8. Find a dentist who buys Halloween candy to send to troops.

- Our orthodontist buys candy each year after Halloween for one dollar per pound to send to the US troops overseas. My kids, along with the neighbors, separate their candy and collectively decide how much to donate. We leave them to their own devices, and we are generally amazed at how much they elect to donate. This can be a great opportunity to discuss donating for those helping our country. It's a lesson about selflessness amid candy hoarding.

9. Exchange the loot.

- The kids can turn in the candy for a present.

- Some parents pay per candy and allow the kids to buy something with the earnings.

10. Make sure they get eight to nine hours of sleep.

- When we sleep, our brains suppress the hunger hormone, ghrelin, so we are less likely to crave sugar. Furthermore, when we sleep, we make more of the hunger-stopping hormone, leptin, which tells the body when it's full and to stop gorging on candy.

- No electronics, including TV and phones, one or two hours before bed. LED lights from electronics prevent kids/teens from falling asleep easily and disrupt their rest all night long.

- Make bedtime the same every night. Keep the amount of post-dinner candy to one or two "fun size" pieces and no more. The sugar and chocolate in the candy will cause disrupted sleep patterns.

Kids should be allowed to keep their Halloween candy for fewer than 5 days.

For my mega list of shopping items from Costco, Walmart, Trader Joe's, Target, Aldi, etc. scan the code for my book resources page.

21

Ho Ho Ho-ld it Together During the Holidays

How to Maintain Health and Weight During the Holiday Season

Once you begin to transition away from the traditional American diet, don't expect your extended family to understand the change. The chemical-packed smorgasbord of holiday food items that are a staple of our holiday meals will not be easily dismissed. I had already annoyed the in-laws by demanding my children get to bed at their scheduled times, but now I was threatening an institution known as Thanksgiving dinner. Gluten free stuffing? Dairy free potato casserole? Organic turkey? I might as well just have recommended we watch Food Inc. rather than football! But I started bringing healthier versions of those beloved dishes and guess what? Last year my dairy free, gluten free, organic buffalo chicken dip won the blind taste test by the naysayers. Little victories.

It seems like every year when holidays roll around, we have the same discussion about sugar, weight gain, skin breakouts, stress, blah blah blah. Let's decide once and for all to stop acting like the holidays are out of our control. It is possible to enjoy the holidays and not feel like you have thrown your health out with the trash.

No Skipping Meals

- Before you go to family dinners where you know there will be an onslaught of cookies, cheese, baked goods, and fried stuff, feed the children fruits and vegetables or an actual meal. Kids who are full are less likely to gorge themselves on junk. Never skip meals to "save up" for the big meal.

Cookie Monsters Beware

- Make a game plan for the number of cookies kids will be permitted to eat at a given destination.

Pace the People

- Make kids play outside or get active in other ways before they can have second helpings.

Fill the Tank

- Have kids drink 6-8 ounces of water with their meal.

Make Fruits and Veggies a Requirement

- If healthy foods aren't eaten, no cookies or baked goods should be allowed. Discuss this rule at home before you leave. Yes, your extended family will make fun of you for this. Those who maintain their weight and stay well during the holidays laugh last.

Count Them

- Allow one cookie per serving of veggies.

Slow Them Down

- Have kids eat with their non-dominant hand.

Walk the Walk

- Take family walks after a big feast. Fresh air will help digestion and the kids will be less crazy. The further we are from food, the less we eat. A walk gives the brain time to realize that the stomach is full.

- Fun fact: It takes about 20 minutes after you start eating for the brain to register that food is entering the stomach.

Never Shame the Kids or Yourself.

Buffet Style

- At buffet tables, walk with the kids around the table first, discuss what to put on the plate and proceed wisely with fruits or veggies on 50% of the plate. It can be done!

Appetizer Table

- Make plates rather than mindlessly eating and picking. A plate provides a great visual for how much you are eating.

Never Shame the Kids or Yourself.

Daily Meals Count

- Thanksgiving is not every day for 30 days in a row. It is one day. Splurge on Thanksgiving, but the rest of the meals that week should be full of veggies, fruits, good proteins and fats. Stay away from sugar. Eat well every day and the splurge day won't be a big deal. One splurge meal is not permission to trash your health for an entire month.

Sugar Quota

- When kids are surrounded by cookies and sugar for the whole holiday season, it is hard to resist. Make certain days dessert days and others non-dessert days. There is no reason to have dessert at every meal. A fun childhood is not defined by sugar.

Don't Be Afraid to Toss

- People are well intentioned, and they want you to feel loved. Welcome their cookie gift, enjoy one or two cookies, and the rest throw in the trash. You are not trashing their love, just the cookies. Your child's skin and your hips will thank you.

Trick the Mind

- For kids who like to overeat at buffets, give them small plates to trick their minds into believing they are eating more food than they truly are.

Self-serve

- Bring a fruit or a veggie option to every occasion. You'll know for sure your kids will have a healthy option to choose from.

No more than 5 food items on that big holiday plate at a time.

For my mega list of shopping items from Costco, Walmart, Trader Joe's, Target, Aldi, etc. scan the code for my book resources page.

22

Leave the Extra Baggage Behind

10 Ways to Prevent Weight Gain on Vacation

Early in my marriage, all road trips started with a stop at the convenience store to stock up on Combos, Hostess Apple Pies, Doritos and Coke. Once we had kids, we simply added stops for Wendy's (which we considered the healthier fast food!) and sometimes for ice-cream. The more our kids annoyed us on a long car ride, the more junk food we would throw into the back seat to quiet them. Then, after fueling them with copious amounts of sugar we were mystified as to why they were screaming out the window at passing vehicles. Even the dog didn't want to sit by them in the car. We now pack as much healthy food as possible into a cooler which not only speeds up our travel time but has also helped our waistlines.

The average person gains between two and seven pounds while on vacation. Weight gain is not the only thing that can be worrisome. There are also the habits that are formed over a short period of time. One week is long enough for most people to give up on exercise and give in to unhealthy eating patterns. These habits and weight gain have been shown to persist for many months after the vacation is over. Don't let this be you!

Here are 10 tips to keep you on track:

1. Remember to pack fruits and veggies.

Problem: While on holiday, most people give themselves permission to indulge in various unhealthy foods. Before anyone realizes it, fries become the standard vegetable at lunch and dinner, ice cream becomes a daily ritual, and mindless snacking permeates beach time.

Solution: Always have washed and cut up fruits and veggies in your cooler for snacking. Fill your belly up with fruits and veggies and then there will be less room for the junk snacks. At restaurants eat a salad or cooked veggies first, before the rest of the meal. Always order salads with dressing on the side. Substitute fruit cups for fries every other night. Pack apples and bananas on day excursions.

2. Cook two of the three daily meals at the apartment or rental home.

Problem: Eating out leads to bigger portions, more fried foods, more dessert, more calories, and more fat, salt, and sugar.

Solution: Go to the local grocery store and stock your apartment or rental home with eggs, fruits, veggies, nitrite free bacon, nitrite free cold cuts, cheese, lettuce, PB, Jelly, oatmeal, etc. Cook a healthy breakfast with protein, complex carbs, and fruits. Pack lunch. Eat out for dinner.

3. Don't underestimate the frozen casserole

Problem: Lots of people hate to cook on vacation. I am one of them.

Solution: If you are traveling locally, prepare one or two casserole dishes ahead of time and freeze. Defrost at your destination. This works great for our beach trips.

4. Watch the drink calories.

Problem: It's easy for kids to indulge endlessly in sodas, sports drinks, juices, milk shakes, etc. For adults, daily alcoholic beverages can add inches to the waist; beer, margaritas, coladas, and daiquiris are high in calories and sugar.

Solution: Always have lots of water on hand. Reserve sugary drinks to once daily. Who wants hyper kids for a week or even a month straight?? Adults should limit their drinks to two per day for several reasons, not just calories. We carry refillable water bottles everywhere we go.

5. Move.

Problem: For most people a week of vacation means a week of parking it in a chair at the beach or mountains and doing nothing.

Solution: Go for a walk on the beach. Rent or bring bikes and go for family bike rides. We went on family sightseeing bike rides through various countries. While marveling at the amazing views, we all got a workout, and no one even noticed. Go hiking, kayaking, paddle boarding, running, surfing, or exploring. Every day do something active for thirty minutes.

6. Protein should be part of all snacks and meals.

Problem: Cereal, crackers, pretzels, chips, toast, and bagels, have a high glycemic index which means these foods cause your blood sugar to spike. When blood sugar spikes quickly, your body makes lots of insulin. With lots of insulin comes a precipitous sugar drop which leads to constant cravings and requests for snacks.

Solution: Pay attention to the foods you eat for breakfast, lunch, dinner, and snacks. Oatmeal breakfast (not the instant kind), eggs, bacon, PBJ, toast with nut butter, etc. will keep blood sugar from spiking and cravings from crashing through your beach read. Packed snacks should include nuts, pistachios, cheese sticks, nut butter dip, rolled up nitrite free cold cuts, or hummus. See more ideas in the snack section.

7. Be mindful of boredom.

Problem: We all get hungry when bored.

Solution: Establish meal and snack times. Don't let the "kitchen" be open endlessly. Sound strange? It will save your ears a lot of whining when you set expectations at the start of the day. This also teaches kids to eat properly when food is available, thus avoiding hunger until the next time the "kitchen" is open for business.

8. Be mindful of thirst.

Problem: Endless caffeinated and sugary beverages and alcohol are dehydrating. Hanging out in hot weather is dehydrating. The body sends hunger signals when it needs water.

Solution: Drinking eight ounces of water dilates the stomach and sends a signal to the brain that eating is in progress. Always have fresh, cold water available. If water is too boring, add slices of lemons, oranges, cucumbers, or mint. Have wedges of watermelon or oranges ready for those who hate water. These fruits have a high water content. I not only carry water at all times, but I also remind all to drink water regularly. There are also apps that remind you to take sips of water and stay hydrated.

9. Be wary of portion sizes at restaurants.

Problem: Not only do we feel we should indulge ourselves constantly while on vacation, but we feel the need to finish the whole plate to get our money's worth.

Solution: Order the entree and have half of it wrapped up to go before it comes to the table. With this technique you can clean the whole plate without worry, and there will be no need for cooking the next day.

10. Be wary of kids' menus.

Problem: Parents assume that kids will only eat pizza, mac and cheese, chicken nuggets, and fries. The kids' menu is the grossest thing at a restaurant. I generally don't even accept one at the table unless it's filled with fun activities to keep boredom at bay.

Solution: Use your travels to explore new places and new foods. Order and share an adult meal. Order half of an adult meal for the kids. If the food is not liked, take it home for leftovers. My pickiest eater managed to find items on the menu that he generally shared with his older sister.

Limit your splurge food items to fewer than 5 per vacay week: such as, funnel cakes, French fries, ice cream, etc.

For my mega list of shopping items from Costco, Walmart, Trader Joe's, Target, Aldi, etc. scan the code for my book resources page.

Pillar II
STRESS

Stress and the Immune System

Stress is a part of everyday life. Some stress is good. It helps us get to school or work on time. It motivates us to finish projects. However, when life surpasses your ability to cope, stress becomes detrimental.

- A systemic review (meta-analysis) of 300 studies showed that chronic stressors, including exam stress, were associated with the suppression of the immune system. Meaning the body produced fewer immune system cells. The fewer cells you have, the more likely you are to get sick from a virus or bacteria. [1]

- Measuring the number of antibodies after the administration of vaccines helps us quantify how the immune system is working. Chronic stress in adults is associated with a poor response to influenza and pneumonia vaccines. [2,3]

- Young adults were experimentally infected with the common cold virus. Those with chronic stress (>1 month) developed cold symptoms more often than those with less stress. [4]

- 334 healthy volunteers were given a shot of rhinovirus, the germ that causes colds, through the nose. Those who had more positive emotions through the day experienced fewer cold symptoms. [5]

- Loneliness and isolation have long been shown to increase stress, thus decreasing the immune system and increasing risk for chronic disease such as obesity, diabetes, heart disease, cancer, and so on. [6]

- People were experimentally given the common cold virus. Those with strong social ties developed fewer colds than those who were socially isolated [7] Being in fairly close proximity to a friend, even a potentially ill one, does not necessarily increase one's own risk for illness. [8]

In summary, the stress from life and all that surrounds COVID-19 puts you and your family at risk to have more significant effects from this notorious viral illness. It also puts you at risk for developing other chronic diseases.

23

Banishing the Burnout

Your Family's Guide to Mindfulness

I used to be a very busy lady, who added 10,000 things to the weekly calendar on a regular basis. I was a ball of stress who felt better in stressful situations. This sounds weird, but stress addiction is a real thing. When we moved to New Zealand, I felt like I was put in Involuntary Stress Rehabilitation. Moving to another country, unplugging from my friends and family, detaching from work, and waiting for a work visa gave me 6 months to detoxify. Breaking the addiction was a highly unpleasant experience. Furthermore, living in the laid-back NZ culture, I realized just how nuts I had become. My year and a half there forced me to reset, declutter, prioritize, and become mindful. I would sometimes hear the kids say, "what does Zen Mom have to say about x, y, or z?"

The modern world has become a difficult place for both adults and children. We're bombarded with expectations, stress, and information every waking moment of the day. Practicing mindfulness is a great way to cut through the daily challenges life throws our way and reduce stress. [1] When we are mindful, we are present in each moment. We check in with our bodies, minds, and surroundings, rather than checking out. Teaching mindfulness to children will give them tools to deal with the ups and downs that life brings. Children will be able to "press pause" rather than react impulsively and thoughtlessly.

Become more mindful to teach mindfulness to your children.

- Develop a mindfulness practice for yourself to teach your children.

- Children learn best by example so model your mindfulness

- Talk to your children as you manage your own stress and emotions, "Mommy is feeling a little stressed right now. Can you help me? Let's take some deep breaths together."

- "Think aloud" to show your children how you speak positively to yourself when you feel nervous. "I'm feeling nervous about giving this presentation at work today. What could I tell myself? I am prepared. I am brave. I can do this."

- If you have a meditation practice, be open about it with your children. Explain that being quiet and still helps calm your mind **Incorporate mindfulness throughout your day.**

- Mornings are generally hectic when trying to get a family out the door. Try to pause together before leaving the house and take 5 calming breaths. This routine does not take much time at all, but it will allow your family to start the day in a better state of mind.

- Bring mindfulness to your drive home. Find a landmark several blocks from your house that will remind you to turn off the radio and drive or ride mindfully the rest of the way home. Aim for 5 minutes of silence.

- Take a listening walk with your children. Listen to the sounds around you, birds, cars, bugs, wind, etc., rather than letting your mind wander. Ask everyone to identify 5 different sounds.

- Eat mindfully. Use your senses to explore and enjoy your food. Talk about the smells, colors, and tastes. No electronics should be present at mealtime.

- Chew your food. Have everyone chew one bite 5 times, the next one 10 times, then the next 20 times. Discuss the differences you notice.

- Start a gratitude practice. Write down or talk about things you are thankful for during dinner or at bedtime.

A great way to be mindful is to "single-task". Today's culture prides itself on multitasking, but people are not really capable of doing more than one thing at the same time. By doing just one task at a time, you will do it better, more mindfully, and even more efficiently!

- Put your phone away while playing with your child.

- Turn off your electronic device when your child or spouse walks into a room after school or in the mornings.

- Help your child with homework after you have cooked dinner, rather than at the same time.

- While getting ready in the morning, choose one task to do at a time.

- Greet your child when you pick him/her up from school. Focus on your child rather than the other parents or your phone.

An excellent meditation tool is the I Spy Jar

- Place uncooked rice and small objects in a jar with a lid

- Make a list of the objects in the jar

- At night to wind down, see if the child can find 10 things in the jar and cross them off the list. The next night look for 10 more until she finds them all

- When your child becomes bored, empty the jar and fill it with new items

- This can also be found on Etsy

Breath Work. Teach your children to breathe properly, and they will learn how to use this powerful tool to calm themselves when they are anxious or upset. If you simply tell kids to breathe deeply, they usually breathe shallowly and rapidly, which is not calming at all! Teach children to breathe in through their noses and to breathe slowly out the mouth, with an emphasis on the exhale. Show them how to do deep belly breathing, rather than shallow chest breathing.

- Tell your child to smell the flower (inhale through nose) and blow out the candle (slow exhale through mouth).

- Have your child hold an imaginary cup of hot chocolate. Smell the hot chocolate (inhale through nose), and then blow on the hot chocolate to cool it down (slow exhale through mouth).

- To help your child breathe into his/her belly, have your child lie down on her back. Place a small stuffed animal on the belly, and have your child try to move the stuffed animal up and down with her breath.

- Try to have your child practice breathing while they are in a good mood so that they can use their breath more easily when they are upset. This is easy to practice when kids are riding in the car.

- Practice regularly for this to be effective. Right before lights out is the easiest time to practice.

Get Outside and Appreciate Weather

- Playing outside is a great way to let children be present and enjoy the moment. Too often, parents are afraid to let children play outside unless the weather is "just right." If it is too cold, too hot, raining, snowing, or windy, parents keep children indoors to protect them.

- Instead of being afraid, use the outdoors as a sensory class-room. Unless there is thunder and lightning, it is probably safe for your child to play outside!

- If it's cold, layer up and go for a walk looking for birds or frozen puddles.

- If it's raining, grab some rain boots and a raincoat, and jump in the puddles or make mud pies!

- If it's hot, turn the sprinklers on or make a slip-and-slide. Fear not, the lawn will recover.

- In the fall, watch for falling leaves and rake them up, then jump in the piles.
- During the day, lay on the grass and talk about cloud shapes. Or walk barefoot in the grass.
- At night, teach the kids about the constellations or listen to the night life.

A grateful mind does not have room for anxiety

- In the morning, start each day with 3 things you are grateful for
- Writing these down helps the mind pay better attention
- Teach your kids this exercise. It can be about anything: I am grateful that it's sunny outside or I am grateful for my dress
- Starting the day with gratitude, sets the stage for a positive day
- Consider ending the day with 3 things you are grateful for

Change the Mindset with The Rule of 5

We all have had days when everything is going splendid. The sun is shining, the homework assignment is turned in on time, the quiz grade is 100%, but a kid on the playground says something mean. Unfortunately, this will ruin the mood and cast a dark shadow on the otherwise beautiful day. This is because our brain is conditioned by evolution to fixate on negative things while discounting the positive things. It is called a negative bias. We not only remember but we will ruminate over negative stimuli 6 times more than the positive ones and this can have an overall impact on our mood, anxiety, and wellbeing. For every negative, come up with 5 positives. Examples:

- If the school day was terrible because a friend did not want to play tag, let your child voice all his frustrations, validate them with empathy. Once he is done explaining his frustration, have him tell you 5 things that were great about the school day

- When siblings squabble and call names, have them come up with 5 nice things as a consequence

- When you get frustrated with one of your kids, come up with 5 things they do to make you smile

Get Mindful with Tapping Mediation

I am not very good at sitting still, quieting my mind, or breathwork. In the past year I have come across a technique and an app that has been life changing. It's called tapping. The app: The Tapping Solution

- In this app you learn how to decrease your state of anxiety and transform yourself into a calm state (think Tasmanian devil transforms to yoga person)

- This practice stimulates the vagus nerve. The vagus nerve connects the brain to the body. It is the counterbalance to the fight or flight system. Low vagal tone leads to stress, anxiety, and depression

- Tapping is a guided therapy, it tells you exactly what to do

- 8-11min duration (generally speaking)

- You can choose from many sessions: Overwhelm, Racing Mind, Sleep Deprivation, COVID worries, IVF, relationships and more

- There are specific kid ones - sleep, school, focus

Call Upon Your Sense of Smell to Calm the Mind

Essential oils are natural products extracted from flowers, leaves, bark or roots of plants. It is best to make sure you use pure essential oils, meaning oils that have not been diluted with chemicals or additives. Calling upon our sense of smell refocuses the mind from anxiety provoking thoughts. There is a strong connection between smell and mood via the part of the brain called the limbic system. In fact, the practice of Aromatherapy evolves around our sense of smell and brain connection.

When in a state of agitation, bad mood, or rumination try the following trick. Have the child pick the smell that she likes the best from the following list. Have her hold the bottle of oil in front of her nose and without touching the oil, have her slowly inhale while saying a positive statement such as "I am strong", "I am brave", "I am calm", "I am a good friend".

- Bergamont[2][3] [7]
- Lavender [4]
- Rose [5]
- Vetiver [6]
- Ylang Ylang [7]
- Chamomille [8]
- Frankincense [9]
- Wild Orange [10][11]
- Grapefruit [11]

There are many ways to bring mindfulness into your family's daily lives. There are no set rules; find out what works best for you and your family and use it. The benefits will exceed your expectations.

End each day with a list of at least 5 things you are grateful for.

For my mega list of shopping items from Costco, Walmart, Trader Joe's, Target, Aldi, etc. scan the code

Pillar III

SLEEP

Sleep and the Immune System

Sleep is a human need. Unfortunately, too many of us place it at the bottom of our priority list. Moreover, the associated stress and human isolation during a pandemic has caused major sleep disruptions for many. There is plenty of data demonstrating a correlation between sleep deprivation and immune system dysfunction.

Let's take a look:

- Research shows that getting fewer than six hours of sleep at night quadruples your chances of getting a cold. [1] Sound familiar, my parents of teens in high school and college? When do they get the most colds? Exam time!

- 60,000 female nurses participated in a study that showed those who slept fewer than 5 hours per night were 1.5 times more likely to develop pneumonia. Interestingly, the same was true for those who slept more than 9 hours per night. [2]

- A study conducted on adult men showed that sleep deprivation decreases your body's response to the flu vaccine. Some subjects were sleep deprived while others slept all night. After they received the flu vaccine, antibodies to the vaccine were measured. Sleep deprived subjects had 50% fewer antibodies than well-rested ones. [3]

- To get a bit nerdier, investigators in Germany dug deeper into sleep and the immune system. They focused on T cells, which are white blood cells critical for immune response. When T cells recognize a target, such as a flu infected cell, they produce sticky proteins, known as integrins, which allow the T cells to attach to the infected cell and kill it. In sleep deprived human subjects, the T cells produce far fewer integrins compared to the well-rested subjects. [4]

In summary:

Less sleep = fewer immune cells + less effective immune cells. Fewer immune cells + less effective immune cells = more sickness. Therefore, less sleep = more sickness.

24

Channel Your Sleeping Beauty

Reclaim Your Night-Time

My favorite activity as an adult is sleeping. I am a sleep-obsessed person. I have a weighted blanket, a cooling mattress pad, and air filtration. My room temperature is specifically set, my bedtime is non-negotiable, and I get very upset when I don't get my full eight hours of beauty rest. If my kids are out late with friends, they must come in and wake me when they get home, which is something that makes them fear for their lives. Allegedly, I come out of sleep swinging. Their new technique is to gently rub my hand and duck. But when I get a good night's sleep, I feel I can conquer the world.

I addressed the importance of sleep for the immune system, now let's discuss how to get that much needed shut eye.

The Role of Melatonin and Sleep

Melatonin is a powerful antioxidant that helps fight inflammation and viral illnesses like Flu and COVID19. [1,2] In the daytime, levels of melatonin are low. As the sun sets, melatonin levels rise which makes us sleepy. When we scroll through Instagram or watch Netflix before bed, the LED lights lower melatonin levels for the night. This prevents us from falling asleep and/or interrupts our sleep all night long (*Figure 1*). Thus, we wake up tired even though we believe we were asleep for 8 hours. Not only is our sleep messed up, but the level of melatonin is not high enough to fight off the germs encountered that day. Moreover, cancer rates have risen dramatically in industrialized nations where screens and artificial light are prevalent. [3] The number one reason for our sleep issues as a culture is artificial light.

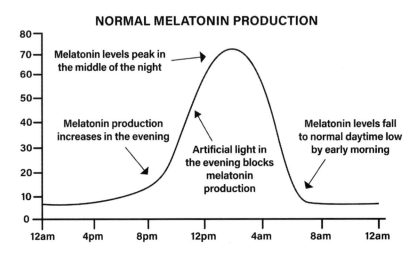

Figure 1

No Phones in Bedrooms (that means parents, too)

Phones on nightstands activate our brains. Harvard Medical School reviewed a great study from JAMA in 2011 about how cell phones activate the brain. Volunteers were placed in a PET scanner with cellphones attached to each ear. Their brain activity was measured when their cellphones were off and then on but muted. Results showed that the brain cells get activated at night when the phones were on. This demonstrates that the brain is stimulated by the energy emitted by phones. [4,5]

Airplane mode is not enough

Cell phones have 4 antennas, Cellular, WIFI, Bluetooth, and Location. When we put our phone in airplane mode, only the cellular signal turns off. This gives us a false sense of security. The best way to prevent the phone from activating our brain at night is to turn it off or charge it in the kitchen. Many are worried about Electric and Magnetic Field (EMF) transmission coming from phones. Turning your device off is the best way to protect yourself from EMF at night. Fun fact: Amazon still sells alarm clocks. Click the QR code below to watch a great 1 Min Pediatric video on sleep.

https://youtu.be/82cvML-FZOk

Teen Sleep

Parents understand the need for sleep in young children. But when it comes to teens, the subject gets a little fuzzy. At this age, things get a bit intense with arguing, the need for control, their need for independence, and so on. Wait this sounds a lot like toddlers... Teens must understand why sleep is important in order for them to make a change. The biggest complaint in clinic from teens: fatigue.

A teenager needs 9-10 hours of sleep per night, minimum. That means going to bed by 9 or 10 p.m. and waking up between 6 and 6:30 a.m. Teenagers go through many growth spurts of their bodies and their brains, and most growth occurs at night during sleep. So, though it may seem annoying, teens need more sleep than adults. The leading cause of fatigue in teens is sleep debt.

Let's do some math based on the 9 hours of sleep the body requires:

Average Weeknight Sleep Duration for Teens in My Practice			
Day	Recommended Hours	Actual Hours	Sleep Deficit
Sunday	9	6	3
Monday	9	6	3
Tuesday	9	6	3
Wednesday	9	6	3
Thursday	9	6	3
Friday	9	12	-3
Saturday	9	12	-3
Totals	63	54	**9 Hours**

9 hours of sleep is not paid back by the time Sunday night arrives. The week begins again. And the sleep debt gets larger which leads to constant fatigue.

What can you do?

- Put electronics away 1 to 2 hours before bed.
- Do not sleep with phones in your room unless you are on-call. Same fun fact: Amazon sells alarm clocks.
- No phones, tablets, or in kids' rooms at night.
- In my house, we all charge our phones in the kitchen in the same drawer. If someone breaks this rule, it results in a 24-hour confiscation of device.
- PARENTS HAVE TO LEAD BY EXAMPLE.

- No TV in kids' bedrooms.

- Don't fall asleep with the TV on.

- If you read on a tablet at night, put it on night mode.

- Blue light-blocker glasses (yellow/red lenses) can make a difference.

- Dim the lights at night. LED lights emit blue light and if your house is too bright at night it can suppress melatonin production.

- Dishes can wait. It took many years of practice for me to let this one go.

- Minimize naps for teens and watch out for long toddler naps.

- Laundry can wait.

- Netflix can wait.

- Kids should have a set bedtime every day of the week. Yes, even on vacation. I understand that occasionally they might stay up late. Occasional does not mean 2-3 times a week.

- Some parents want to have their young kids sleep later in the morning, so they keep them up later at night. This most often fails and leads to cranky kids because a child's circadian rhythm is more like that of a rooster.

- Keep the house temperature cool at night. Cool temps cue the body to slow down and prepare for sleep. Room temps between 60 and 67 degrees Fahrenheit are optimal for sleeping. Temperatures above 75 or below 54 degrees interfere with sleep. [6]

- Do homework/work with your phone on "do not disturb" mode. Fact: every time you interrupt your work to check out a text, it takes you 7 to 10 minutes to get back on task. This can add up quickly.

Pro Tip
Set a time each night for the entire family to turn in all phones and other devices. No devices in bedrooms.

Suggested Sleep Requirements	
Age	Sleep Requirements per 24 hours
0-2 months	12-18 hours
3-11 months	14-15 hours
1-3 years	12-14 hours
3-5 years	11-13 hours
5-10 years	10-11 hours
10-17 years	8.5-9.25 hours
Adults	7-9 hours

Make sure you get a good night's sleep at least 5 times per week.

For my mega list of shopping items from Costco, Walmart, Trader Joe's, Target, Aldi, etc. scan the code for my book resources page.

Pillar IV
MOVEMENT

Movement and the Immune System

One of the many differences between plants and humans, is that humans have the ability to move. However, many of us living in modernized societies have become rooted to our chairs and implanted on our couches. The lack of movement has caused our bodies to wilt and our health to rot. It is essential for the human frame to move. It makes the heart pump more efficiently, bacteria and viruses are flushed out of our airways and lungs, antibodies and white blood cells circulate more rapidly, the core body temperature rises, and this reduces the number of viruses/bacteria circulating in the body.

Lastly, exercise decreases stress hormone levels. Elevated hormone levels, such as cortisol, are directly linked with more colds, viruses, and even cancer. (Think final exams, huge presentations, and managing small children all day) [9]

Several studies have shown that moderate exercise (30-60 minutes in duration) reduces the risk of infections, such as cold and flu:

- Those who moderately exercise 3-4 times a week have 50% fewer sick days than those who do nothing and are sedentary. [1]

- A study of 1,000 people found that staying active nearly halved the odds of catching cold viruses and for those who got a cold, it made the infection less severe. [2]

- 45 minutes of brisk walking 5 times per week has been associated with increased numbers of Natural Killer Cells and decreased episodes and severity of the common cold. [3]

- Having sex once or twice a week was shown to boost secretory IgA which protects the body from cold and flu. [4]

- Moderate exercise increases the number of white blood cells such as neutrophils, natural killer cells and lymphocytes, and it enhances their killing abilities. [5,6]

- Light to moderate physical activity decreases the risk of death from the flu. [7]

- Interestingly, overtraining (intense activity over 75min) results in decreased number of lymphocytes, natural killer cells, secretory IgA, and neutrophils. Competitive athletes suffer from more colds and viral illnesses than non-athletes. [5,8]

25

They've Got to Move it Move it

Kids and Exercise

When my kids were in Elementary School, they took a bus to school, which was a mile from our house. On my day off, each Friday, I made it my mission to walk my kids to school instead. Initially it was just the four of us, then another family joined in, and before long more kids from the bus stop were walking with us. Pretty soon we had an entire gang in tow. We even ordered T-shirts and called ourselves the Fun Friday Fitness Group.

The average American child spends five to eight hours a day in front of a digital screen. That was the number before virtual school became the norm. Isn't it interesting that in today's world we must have a chapter in a book about how to get kids to play outside? We have become an indoor and sedentary society. To be blunt, we sit on our butts too much. Here are some reasons kids don't get enough outdoor playtime:

We are concerned about the weather:

- We fret over the weather app - it's too cold, too hot, too windy, too rainy, or too sunny.

- Without realizing it, we use a lot of negative intonations about the great outdoors.

- Kids become wary and uncomfortable about the thought of how cold or hot they will be.

- Send kids outside. Most of us live in temperate zones. They will be fine with appropriate clothes and hydration.

- I often encounter kids who can't play outside in 29 degree weather due to the cold, but they ski at fancy resorts without issue when the thermometer registers 3 degrees.

We get stressed that they might get dirty:

- They should get dirty and messy. That's what kids do.

- Grass stains might not come out of clothes – no big deal.

- My favorite kids are those who come to the office with sand in their shoes, mulch in their pants, bruised legs from climbing too many things, and dirt under their fingernails.

We are afraid they will get hurt.

- It's much safer being inside on the iPad, or so we think.

- Kids are supposed to explore the world, fall down, break bones, get stitches, bruise, bleed and so on. It's okay.

- In New Zealand, the school principal pulled me aside to let me know that kids there are allowed to climb trees on the playground and that sometimes they fall out of trees and break bones. I looked at her puzzled. Then I realized that once she heard my American accent, she assumed I was afraid of my kids getting hurt.

We are worried that our children will be abducted.

- Kidnappings make headlines, but abductions are rare.

- Fewer than 350 people under the age of 21 have been abducted by strangers in the United States per year between 2010 and 2017.

- The federal government estimated about 50,000 people under the age of 18 years old, were reported missing in 2001.

- Only about 100 cases per year can be classified as abductions by strangers. [1]

We are petrified about child trafficking. [2, 3]

- The majority of children are trafficked by someone they know.

- The average age of victims is 14-16yrs old.

- This doesn't happen with a snatching from the front yard. Perpetrators recruit their victims over time.

- Recruitment occurs most often at schools, bus stations, homeless shelters, malls, and on the Internet.

We are scared that they will be bored and whine a lot.

- Kids are supposed to be bored and bother the adults.

- Out of boredom comes creativity.

- Kids complain because they can't rule the world. No one cares.

- They should go outside whether they like it or not.

- The iPad is easy, they are mesmerized. They don't have to be creative because the iPad apps do it for them.

- My boys like to watch other people play video games. How lazy is that? They are not even playing the game; they are watching others do it. I don't get it.

We fear missing Instagram and Facebook updates:

- Let's face it. We are as addicted as the kids are to electronic devices.

- If our kids are outside, we must monitor them, thus we can't fully focus on the latest messages on IG or FB.

- It is much easier to have the youngsters on their own devices so we can get our fix.

The recommended time for physical activity per day is 60 minutes. However, studies have shown benefits from just 30 minutes of activity in adults. The first step:

Turn off Electronics.

When my kids were younger, I struggled with getting them to play outside. So, I made up a rule. They were only able to watch as much screen time as the time they spent outside. Thus, for every one minute of outside playtime, they earned one minute of screen time. No outside time, then no screen time that day. They managed to play outside no matter the weather almost every day.

Physical activity does not need to be complicated and can include:

- 30 minutes of walking (walk your kids to school).
- 30 minutes of biking (bike with the kids to school).
- A few laps in the pool, or just playing in the pool.
- Taking stairs instead of the elevator, especially when it's only one floor.
- Exploring parks - print out a map and make it your family's mission to go to all the playgrounds and rate them. My kids loved discussing the pros and cons of various excursions.
- Buy chalk and bring back old school games (hopscotch, 4 corners, etc.).
- Have an art competition with chalk or sand.
- Print out a list of outdoor things they need to find and call it a treasure hunt (there are tons of ideas on Pinterest).
- Sticks and sheets make great forts.
- Ride bikes, scooters, or skateboards.
- Jump rope.

- Play soccer, basketball, badminton, or football.
- Play tag, hide-and-go seek, red light, green light.
- Family walks are so great to relax, talk about the day, and reduce everyone's stress.
- Make mud pies and mud castles.
- Catch bugs.
- Plant a garden.
- Dig holes and bury things.
- Play with water - tables, slip and slides, or kiddie pools.

The Virtual School Dilemma

This turn of events made my kids more sedentary. My solution:

- Our entire family got Fitbits. Everyone took at least 10,000 steps per day to have access to phones, iPads, or Xboxes after school was done for the day.
- If 10,000 steps were not achieved by the time I went to bed, I took all non-school devices away. I had to follow through with consequences and it was awful. But it worked. It only had to happen once in my house and the message was received. No yelling or nagging required.

Make sure your kids play outside more than 5 days per week.

For my mega list of shopping items from Costco,
Walmart, Trader Joe's, Target, Aldi, etc. scan the code for
my book resources page.

Pillar V

ENVIRONMENT

Environment and the Immune System

There are more than 85,000 toxic chemicals in our daily environment. [1] These include cosmetics, cookware, plastics, sunscreen, cleaners, and so on. The FDA does not require manufacturers of cosmetics, cleaners, detergents, etc. to list their ingredients. What's even more distressing is that the FDA's regulations are lax compared to the European Union (EU) or any other country in the world. For example, as of 2013 the EU has banned 1,328 chemicals from cosmetics, while the US has only banned 11. [2]

Most of the time we have no idea what we are using. We only have marketing as our guide. For those of us trying to clean up our environment, the number of choices is overwhelming. But, before you chuck this book at the wall, I have some great news. The following chapters will have lists of ingredients, and details about ingredients and illness, but at the end of each chapter you will have a handy dandy tip to make your life so much easier and cleaner. You are welcome!

There are many things in our environment that have been shown to depress our immune system and put us at risk for viral illnesses, cancer, and other chronic diseases. Out of the 85,000 toxins I chose 5 to illustrate my point about the immune system.

- A study of 9000 children in Europe showed a correlation between the use of bleach products and viral illnesses. In homes where bleach was used at least once a week, the kids had higher rates of influenza and recurrent tonsillitis. [3]

- In a different study, "Women cleaning at home or working as occupational cleaners had accelerated decline in lung function, suggesting that exposures related to cleaning activities may constitute a risk to long-term respiratory health." [4]

- Triclosan has been used in antibacterial soaps since the 1970's. Studies show that higher triclosan urine levels in kids were associated with more hay fever symptoms and allergies. [5] In the same study, higher urinary levels of Bisphenol A (BPA) in kids were associated with a depressed immune system. Where do you find BPA? In plastic for starters.

- Teflon is a nonstick agent on cookware has been linked to immune system dysfunction, thyroid issues, and cholesterol abnormalities in

- children. The findings were based on a study evaluating 69,000 people. [6]

- Perfluorinated compounds (PFC) are found in Teflon. High blood levels of PFC's in children were found to correlate with decreased antibody production after vaccines. [7]

- Phthalates are found in food, leached from plastics, household cleaners, sunscreens, etc. A study of 300 inner-city children, showed that prenatal exposure to phthalates increased the children's risk of developing asthma. [8]

26

Here Comes the Sun

Choosing the Best Protection for our Skin

I grew up lathering my body in baby oil to cook my skin and maximize my tan. My husband is genetically incapable of applying sunscreen correctly when he occasionally decides to put some on. Suffice it to say we were not role model parents to teach our children about the harmful effects of the sun. It wasn't until I began to see the aging effects of the sun on my own skin that I began to emphasize the importance of sun protection. Soon after, I also started considering the chemicals used in the products made to protect us. My children, unfortunately, have often been the guinea pigs in my trials of sun protection products and more than once have ended up looking like ghosts or running from the burning spray in their eyes. I continue to search for the holy grail of all sunscreens: an SPF Snowsuit!

Many people assume that sunscreen goes on top of your skin and stays there. No big deal, right? It actually is a big deal because the skin is a living organ. In fact, it is the largest organ in the body. When we apply anything to our skin, it penetrates through the skin cell layers and it reaches the capillaries (tiny vessels in the skin). The product components move through the walls of the blood vessels and the blood carries the ingredients to other parts of the body. Think morphine patches, birth control patches, and ADHD medication patches. Drug companies understand that chemicals can be applied to the skin and distributed to organs. We should too. Sunscreen can be full of toxic chemicals. It may reduce our chances of skin cancer but can cause other health problems.

The FDA has raised concerns over the ingredients in sunscreen. It has put the entire industry on alert because we only have enough safety information on two out of sixteen sunscreen ingredients: zinc oxide and titanium dioxide. This is not very reassuring since we have been lathering ourselves with all the other chemicals for years. As I said, for years I used baby oil and competed for the best tan. Not my smartest moments.

Ingredients to Avoid and Why

Before we get down to the nitty gritty, let's discuss the EWG. They are the Environmental Working Group, a non-profit, non-partisan organization dedicated to protecting human health and the environment. They score products based on safety data. EWG rates ingredients from 0-10, with 0 being the cleanest and 10 the worst.

Oxybenzone (EWG 8)

- This dangerous sunscreen chemical has been detected in nearly every American in random testing.
- FDA found blood levels 438 times above cutoff for systemic exposure.
- Found in mothers' milk after sunscreen exposure.
- 1% to 9% skin penetration in lab studies.
- Correlation with lower testosterone levels in men and boys.
- Correlations with lower sperm counts and abnormal sperm quality.
- Increases risk for endometriosis.
- Is associated with altered birth weight in human studies.
- Has high risk of skin allergy. [1]

Octinoxate (EWG 6)

- Found in mother's milk after sunscreen exposure.
- FDA found blood levels 13 times above cutoff for systemic exposure.
- Exhibits activity similar to estrogen and thyroid hormone.
- Animal studies showed alterations in their reproductive system, thyroid gland and behavioral issues.
- Has moderate risk of skin allergy. [2]

Homosalate (EWG 4)

- Found in mother's milk after sunscreen exposure.
- FDA found blood levels 37 times above cutoff for systemic exposure.
- Disrupts estrogen, androgen and progesterone production.
- This chemical also breaks down into other smaller components which may damage the body. [3]

Octisalate (EWG 3)

- Widespread use and stabilizes avobenzone.
- FDA study found blood levels 10 times above cutoff for systemic exposure.
- Low risk of skin allergy. [4]

Octocrylene (EWG 3)

- Widespread use.
- Found in mother's milk after sunscreen exposure.
- FDA study found blood levels 14 times above cutoff for systemic exposure.
- Low risk of skin allergy. [5]

Avobenzone (EWG 2)

- Widespread use.

- Best UVA filter for non-mineral sunscreens.

- Unstable in sunshine – must be mixed with stabilizers.

- Found in mother's milk after sunscreen exposure.

- FDA study found blood levels 14 times above cutoff for systemic exposure.

- High rates of skin allergy. [6]

Parabens (EWG score not available)

- A group of related chemicals commonly used as preservatives in cosmetic products.

- Prevent the growth of bacteria and mold in products.

- The most common parabens in beauty products are butylparaben, ethyl paraben, methylparaben, and propylparaben.

- They mimic the activity of estrogen in the body. Studies show a link between increased urinary levels and decreased fertility. Women who had elevated levels in their urine levels were more likely to have preterm births.

- Adolescent girls who wear makeup every day were found to have 20 times the levels of propylparaben in their urine compared to those who never or rarely wear makeup. The use of body and face lotions, hair products, sunscreens and makeup have all been predictors of and correlated with remarkably increased levels of urinary parabens. [7,8,9,10]

Phthalates (EWG score not available)

- Appear as "fragrance" or Dibutyl phthalate (DBP) on the label of sunscreens.

- Chemicals that make plastic more flexible; these were previously present in children's toys but have recently been banned.

- Have been shown to lower levels of testosterone.

- Are associated with abnormal urogenital anatomy of boys called "Phthalate Syndrome".

- Are associated with increased risk for PCOS. [11]

Retinal Palmitate (EWG score not available)

- A form of vitamin A.

- Has been shown, when applied topically, to react with UV rays, increasing the risk of skin tumors in hairless mice.

- No data shown in humans; however, the European Scientific Committee on Consumer Safety remains concerned and at this time this ingredient is not permitted in European Sunscreens.

- Avoid the following: retinol, retinyl palmitate, retinyl acetate and retinyl linoleate. [12]

Lowest Risk Ingredients

- Zinc Oxide (EWG 2)

- Titanium Dioxide (EWG 2)

- Avobenzone (EWG 2)

How to choose a sunscreen:

- Choose a mineral-based product. These contain zinc oxide and/or titanium dioxide as the active ingredients.

- Pick a product with an SPF between 15- 50. According to the FDA, products with higher SPFs are inherently misleading, and could encourage people to stay in the sun too long.

- Avoid spray products to reduce inhalation concerns. Choose lotions or creams instead.

- Reapply sunscreen often: at least every two hours, and more frequently if you get in water or towel off.

- Remember that sunscreen is just one part of sun protection. It's important to wear hats, sunglasses, and shirts. Find or make your own shade and avoid peak midday sun.

But wait, before you lose your mind trying to remember all the ingredients to avoid, let me make your life a little easier. Let's talk about the Think Dirty App.

https://www.thinkdirtyapp.com/

- Download the app using the QR scanner above.
- Enter the name of your sunscreen in search box.
- Note the number on the right side. That's the rating: 0-10.

10 is toxic. 0 is squeaky clean.

- Click on the product to find out why it has that specific rating.
- The ingredients will be listed and color coded depending on concern level.
- Click on the ingredient to get details on the health impacts.
- If your product is 5 or more, click on "Our Picks" to get a list of clean products.

My Favorite Sunscreens	
Alba Botanicals Mineral Sunscreen*	Babo Botanicals Sheer Zinc
Badger	BARE
Beautycounter	Coola Mineral
Goddess Garden	Supergoop Mineral Sunscreen Mist
Thinksport adult/baby	

*Product I currently use

ProTip:
Even health-conscious companies may have some clean and some dirty products. Check each product's rating individually. There are many options out there; these are just a few suggestions.

Use sunscreens rated less than 5 on the Think Dirty App.

For my mega list of shopping items from Costco, Walmart, Trader Joe's, Target, Aldi, etc. scan the code

27
Stop Bugging Me
Everything You Have Ever Wanted to Know About Bug Spray

We used to live in Los Angeles, where there were no bugs. Zero. My kids played on their cement patio without a worry. One year later we moved to NC. The day we moved into our new house we sent the kids out to play in our yard full of grass and flowers. Within 30 seconds they came into the house screaming "BUUUUGGGSSSS". Really??? Three years later when my youngest was 2 years old, we realized that he was the perfect mosquito snack. His siblings would go on search and rescue missions to save him from the pesky bugs. He would have as many as 20 on his face alone. The only thing that would prevent this bloodletting was DEET. But there was no way I was going to spray this tiny human with that stuff daily, or multiple times a day for that matter. Thus, the search for a less toxic bug spray ensued.

During spring and summer as mosquitoes and ticks swarm, so do the latest bug repellent companies and products claiming to keep them at bay. I would love to use the Think Dirty App to keep this simple, but in the case of bug sprays things are a little more complicated.

For those who live in a high-risk area for Lyme disease:

- Wear lightweight, summer friendly clothes with long sleeves, pants, socks, and close-toed shoes when spending time outdoors.
- Wear light colored clothing to spot tics.
- Keep lawn at a low level.

- Avoid woodpiles where small furry critters like to hang out.

- Enclose the yard to prevent deer from entering.

- Spray your yard with natural anti-tick and mosquito spray.

- Get an outdoor cat that hunts (we had one named Oreo who got rid of all the wildlife in our yard. Unfortunately, birds were victims too).

Rates of insect-borne illnesses are on the rise, and some, like Lyme, are very debilitating. As much as I would like to only recommend the use of essential oils on children, we need to consider the effectiveness as well as safety/toxicity of bug spray ingredients. The 2 establishments I trust to help me sort through the vast amount of data, are the EWG and Environmental Protection Agency (EPA). We have talked about EWG, but what is the EPA? This is a federal government agency that regulates the manufacturing, processing, distribution, and use of chemicals and other pollutants. Ideally you want to use an EPA registered repellent.

The **Top 5 Active Ingredients** in bug sprays recommended and evaluated by EWG and EPA:

- DEET

- Picaridin

- IR3535

- Oil of Lemon Eucalyptus

- 2-Undecannone

DEET

- Aim for <30%

- The safety data on DEET depends on concentration and exposure time.

- It has been around for 60 years.

- Concentrations indicate how long the repellents last, not how effective it is. Concentrations higher than 50% have not been shown to be more effective. The CDC recommends using concentrations <10% in no known disease risk area and <30% in a known disease risk area. In children, see the table below and discuss with your doctor.

- It may dissolve or damage plastics.

- Neurotoxicity has been demonstrated in animals, but studies did not show young children to be at an increased risk. [1]

- Another study in 2018 showed DEET to be of low toxicity to humans and that any side effects were a result of spraying on the lips and mouth, and/or in high concentrations. [2]

- Other issues identified: A review by the CDC found that neurological issues from DEET occurred in those with high exposure (park rangers who applied DEET in spray or lotion many times throughout the day), those who used very high concentration of DEET (30-100%), and people who ingested DEET.[3]

- People who used DEET daily reported rashes, dizziness, difficulty concentrating, and headaches. [4]

If you must use DEET

- Spray clothing (rather than skin) and allow it to dry, then dress.

- Shower kids as soon as you come in from outside.

- Never use sunscreen with bug-repellent combos.

- Do not spray hands or faces, around mouth or eyes, on cuts, wounds, or irritated skin.

- Do not let kids under 10 years old self-apply.

- Do not spray near food or eating utensils. As a rule, don't spray the kids. Spray your hands and apply to children.

- Wash hands after application.

- Wash treated clothing before wearing it again.

Follow These Guidelines from Health Canada [5]

Age	Recommendations
0 to 6 months	No DEET
6 to 24 months	5-10% DEET Use only when bug risks are high Limit to one application per day
2 to 12 years	5-10% DEET Limit to three applications per day Avoid prolonged use
General population	No more than 30% DEET allowed in products

*One exception: According to the EWG, if you're using DEET to protect kids in an area known for ticks carrying Lyme disease or Zika outbreaks, a concentration of 20% to 30% may be appropriate. Check with your doctor.

Picaridin

- Aim for <20%.

- Found by EWG to be as effective as DEET, without the neurotoxicity concerns.

- A 2018 science review found no significant difference in performance between Picaridin and DEET. [6]

- At a concentration of 20%, it is effective against mosquitoes and ticks for 8-14 hours, and at a concentration of 10% it is effective for 5-12 hours. [7]

- Picaridin does not carry the same neurotoxicity concerns as DEET.

If you must use Picaridin

- Use the same precautions as DEET.

IR3535

- 3-[N-Butyl-N-acetyl]-aminopropionic acid.

- Aim for less than 20%.

- Can be irritating to eyes but poses few other safety risks.

- May dissolve or damage plastics.

- Similar or slightly less effective than DEET and picaridin against mosquitoes. [8]

- Provides over twice the protection time of DEET, picaridin or Oil of Lemon Eucalyptus against deer ticks. [8]

- Found in combination sunscreens and repellent. Never purchase these because sunscreens should be applied every 2 hours which will increase the risk of toxicity from this repellant.

Oil of Lemon Eucalyptus

- Extract of the eucalyptus tree native to Australia. The tree extract is refined to intensify the concentration of the naturally occurring substance PMD (*para*-menthane-3,8-diol) from 1-65%. There is also synthetic PMD.

- PMD has a 2hr duration of protection against ticks and mosquitoes according to the EPA.

- Oil of Lemon Eucalyptus appears to last longer and be more effective than synthetic PMD.

- The CDC warns against the use in children less then 3yrs old since we don't have enough safety data. [9]

2-Undecannone

- Can be found naturally in many plants such as cloves, strawberries and tomatoes.

- In lab studies, this did not show toxicity with oral ingestion, but it did show risk for skin and eye irritation.

- The only product available is Bite Blocker BioUD. It is registered to provide 5 hours of mosquito repellence and 2 hours of tick protection.

- It appears to be as effective as DEET. [10]

Recommended Insect Repellents		
DEET	**Picaridin**	**Oil of Lemon Eucalyptus**
Ben's Tick and Insect Repellent (30% DEET)	Natrapel (20% Picaridin)	Murphy's Naturals*
Sawyer Family Insect Repellent Lotion (encapsulated 20% DEET)	OFF! FamilyCare Insect Repellent II Spritz (5% Picaridin)	Cutter Lemon Eucalyptus
Off! Insect Repellent Family Care Fragrance Free (DEET 7%)	Sawyer (20% Picaridin)	Repel Plant Based Lemon Eucalyptus

*The spray I use on my family

 Familiarize yourself with the 5 ingredients effective against ticks and mosquitoes.

For my mega list of shopping items from Costco, Walmart, Trader Joe's, Target, Aldi, etc. scan the code for my book resources page.

28

The Dirty on Keeping Clean

How to Choose Soaps, Lotions, Detergents, Cleaners and Potions

My house was a chemically laden cesspool. The common response to chicken juice dripping on the counter was Clorox. Dirty coolers were cleaned with bleach. Laundry was not considered clean unless it smelled of bleach or Tide. Let's not forget the aromatic plugins I used regularly. We demanded and expected clean to have a smell. Over the years, our use of chemicals lessened, but the complaints increased: why does my clean shirt smell like shirt? How can you be sure that soap and water removes chicken bacteria? Why did the scented candles go away? They gave meaning to my life. My people have been known to bring Tide into the house and wash their laundry on the down-low with the contraband while I am at work. Though I disapprove of said detergent, I choose to applaud self-sufficiency in the laundry department.

When it comes to this category things can be so confusing. The FDA does not require the industries producing cosmetic or household cleaning products to put the ingredients on the label. And when they do put some of the ingredients on the label, what are those ingredients anyway? Most of us are not chemical engineers, after all.

Did you know that the European Union has banned over 1300 chemicals from cosmetics and in the US, we've only banned 11? Did you know that in the US, we test new chemicals that are introduced to the market, but chemicals previously approved without any data are not subjected to the same scrutiny? [1]

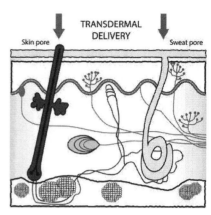

Cosmetics get absorbed through the largest organ, the skin. Right under the skin, there are vessels. When the lotion is put on the skin, it penetrates through the epidermis and it is absorbed into the blood vessels, bypassing the liver. The liver is the great detoxifier of the body. Thus, when we eat chemicals, the liver is hard at work getting rid of these unwanted toxins from the body. When synthetics encounter our skin, they get absorbed and travel freely throughout the body.

Chemicals in our environment, such as cleaners and detergents, can be inhaled, eaten, or absorbed into the skin. When we bleach our countertops, the chemical, bleach, remains on the surface and when we prep our food on that counter, it is then transferred to the food and to the person eating it.

The various chemicals in our cleaners and cosmetics have been implicated in allergic reactions, respiratory problems, cancer, and endocrine dysfunction such as low sperm count, thyroid issues, etc.

Here is a brief list of ingredients to avoid

- Parabens
- Phthalates
- Artificial fragrance and parfum
- Sodium Lauryl Sulfate
- Polyethylene Glycol
- Toluene
- Formaldehyde

- Triclosan

- Diethanolamine

I can go into tons of details about what they cause, where you find these, and the alternatives but that would take up an entire book. Instead, we are going to use THE RULE OF 5 to simplify your life and give the *Think Dirty App* a little love again.

As I discussed before, *Think Dirty* is an app that educates the consumer on the ingredients in products and teaches people how to shop for cosmetics, soaps, lotions, detergents, and cleaners. They have investigated thousands of brands and over one million products to make your life easier.

https://www.thinkdirtyapp.com/

- Download the app > QR

- Type in your product or scan the bar code.

- Think Dirty will rate your product on a scale from 0-10.

- 0 = super clean 10 = super dirty.

- Select the product to get the details of the ingredients and how they measure up.

- Click on the ingredients individually to learn more.

- If the product rating is less than 5, you are good to go.

- If your product is 5 or higher, you can click on the product, then click on "our favorites" at the top of page.

The following is what I currently use in my house. These are not the only great products; they are just what work for my family.

Our Current Products	
Hand Soap	Branch Basics*
Disinfectant for all surfaces	Force of Nature*
Counter Tops	Norwex, Polly Clean Cloth,* Branch Basics*
Stainless Steel	Norwex
Mirrors	Norwex Window Cloth
Floors	Hot water and vinegar, Norwex Mop
Dish Detergent/Soap	Seventh Generation Free and Clear
Laundry Detergent	Seventh Generation, Branch Basics
Armpit stains	Hydrogen peroxide mixed with baking soda
Smelly clothes	1 cup of vinegar in the wash
Good Smelling Laundry	Grow Fragrance (100% plant based)
Brighten Whites	½ to 1 cup hydrogen peroxide per load, Molly Suds, Mrs. Stewart's Liquid Bluing

*Items with which I am affiliated and use in my home and office

Make sure your products are rated less then 5 on the Think Dirty App.

For my mega list of shopping items from Costco, Walmart, Trader Joe's, Target, Aldi, etc. scan the code for my book resources page.

29

Fluorination Station

The Fluoride Debate Clarified

The other day I looked at my 13-year-old son's yellow teeth and asked him a question he appeared to have never heard before, "Did you brush your teeth today?" He looked appalled and said, "You never reminded me!" WHAAAATT? First of all, he is 13 years old. We could stop there but let me do the math for your entertainment. 2 x 365 days of the year for 10 years = 7,300 times I have asked him this question. Of note, this is a low estimate because I generally repeat myself multiple times daily. In his case, an overexposure of fluoride does not seem likely.

Despite the popular belief that fluoridation of water reduces the incidence of cavities in kids, it has long been a very controversial topic. I have struggled with this topic my entire medical career. I have tortured dentists, colleagues, and parents trying to better understand the subject and come up with solutions. After tons of research, I have come to several conclusions and recommendations.

The History of Water Fluoridation:

- In 1945, Grand Rapids, Michigan, became the first community in the world to add fluoride to tap water. This was based on observational work that naturally occurring fluoride in the water systems may reduce cavities. Since 1945, this has been discussed as one of the greatest accomplishments of the 20th Century.

- As of 2001, the CDC reviewed data on the effectiveness of fluoride and dental cavities. They found 3 things with enough evidence for cavity protection:
  - food
  - topical fluoride
  - dental sealants

There is not enough evidence for oral fluoride supplements or fluoridated water. [1]

- In 2012, Harvard School of Public Health (HSPH) and China Medical University in Shenyang, did a meta-analysis of 27 studies and found a strong correlation between water fluoridation and abnormal neurological development. However, there were many confounders and the levels of fluoride in the studies were much higher than in the US. [2]

- In 2015, The Cochrane Collaboration, looked at 155 studies and found insufficient evidence to determine whether water fluoridation decreases cavities in children. Out of all the studies reviewed, none had adequate information to determine the effectiveness of fluoride on cavity prevention in adults. [3]

- In the latest publication by JAMA Pediatrics, reviewed by David C. Bellinger, PhD, MSc, from Boston Children's Hospital, Harvard Medical School, a link was shown between maternal fluoride exposure and a decrease in children's IQ. I am highlighting this specific article because it was a gamechanger in my medical practice. Let's take a closer look:

JAMA Pediatrics Aug 19, 2019 [4]

- 512 mother-child pairs from Canada were recruited during pregnancy and followed until the kids were 3-4 years of age.

- At 3 points during pregnancy, the moms had their urinary fluoride concentrations measured.

- Children's IQs were assessed at 3 and 4 years old.

Conclusions:

- Women living in areas with water fluorination had higher levels of fluoride in their urine.
- For each 1mg/L of fluoride in urine there was an associated drop of 4.5 IQ points in boys.
- For every 1mg of ingested fluoride there was an associated drop of 3.5 IQ points for both girls and boys.

What to Do

- Pregnant mamas, please drink spring water. Pour it into glass bottles.
- Use spring water for mixing baby formulas.
- Pregnant mamas don't brush your teeth with fluorinated toothpaste.
- Filter your water. See below.
- Do not panic. The goal is not to eliminate all fluoride, which is hard to do. The goal is to reduce our exposure while protecting our brain and teeth.
- The body is able to detoxify (get rid of toxins) with the right tools. For example, eating a diet full of vegetables creates alkaline urine, which results in more fluoride being excreted. Conversely, a diet high in meat leads to more acidic urine, thus less fluoride being excreted. [5]
- Fluoride is naturally occurring in the environment and some foods: [6]
  - 3.5oz of black tea = 0.25-0.39mg
  - 5oz of white wine = 0.3mg
  - 3.5oz of canned crab = 0.21mg
  - Russet baked potato with skin on = 0.14mg

Water Filtration

- Carbon filters are not effective. Brita or faucet-mounted filters do not remove fluoride.

- Don't assume that your whole house water filtration system removes 99% of fluoride. Most do not.

- Make sure the product you choose has been third party tested to verify their claims.

My Favorite Water Filtration Brands	
Water Pitcher	Clearly Filtered
Counter Top Filter	Aqua Tru*
Water Bottles	Clearly Filtered
In Line Fridge Filters	Clearly Filtered
Shower Filter	Clearly Filtered
Reverse Osmosis	1. iSpring RCC7AK-UV Reverse Osmosis 75GPD*
	2. Home Master TMJRF2-BK Jr F2 Reverse Osmosis
	3. APEC Essence ROES-50 Reverse Osmosis Filter

*Items with which I am affiliated and use in my home and office

Dental Care

- Juice, soda, sport drinks, fruit pouches, candy, cookies, gummies, processed foods, fast food, nighttime bottles, chocolate milk, and breakfast cereal all contribute to cavities.

- In our society we have been using fluoride in our water to counteract the horrid dental effects of the American diet!!!

- Topical fluoride varnish on teeth is a cavity protectant and the kids generally do not swallow significant quantities. Varnish goes on the teeth where it is needed, as opposed to fluoride in water, which goes to all body parts.

- Dental sealants are protective, but then we get into the plastic issue.

- Obviously, brush and floss the kids' teeth.

- No fluoride supplements.

- See your dentist at least twice a year to assess for cavities and ask her/him about the best approach for your children.

Consider Hydroxyapatite

Enamel is the hardest substance in the body; however, it is under daily attack by plaque and acid formed by our modern diet. The substance that gives enamel its strength is hydroxyapatite, aka HA, which forms a unique crystal structure that makes up 97% of enamel, 70% of dentin, and 60% of our bones. [7]

Hydroxyapatite (HA) in toothpaste:

- Helps to rebuild tooth structure without any known side effects. [8]

- HA is absorbed down to the root of the tooth. This is most beneficial for tooth decay because HA can reach down into the furthest area of decay to rebuild enamel on any tooth surface. [9,10]] Studies show that this compound reduces the size of cavities. [11,12]]

- 10% hydroxyapatite has been shown to be as effective as fluoride in preventing dental carries in children. [13]

- It decreases tooth sensitivity and makes teeth whiter.[14]

- Using HA toothpaste will help protect your teeth from "acid attacks" by bacteria, but without wrecking your oral microbiome. Fluoride, on the other hand, is bactericidal and tends to kill off bacteria in the mouth.

- Preliminary studies show it may help with gum disease. [15]

I currently use RiseWell toothpaste, though the family is not yet on board with me. It's great for kids of all ages, even the littles that swallow toothpaste. The other toothpaste on the market is BOKA. I have not tried it yet.

 Remember the 5 F's: Fresh veggies, Filtered water, Floss and brush, Find a new toothpaste, Fluoride varnish for those at risk for cavities.

For my mega list of shopping items from Costco, Walmart, Trader Joe's, Target, Aldi, etc. scan the code for my book resources page.

30

Life with Plastic, Not Fantastic

Understanding the Dangers of Plastics

Plastic is everywhere. It's easy, cheap, and it doesn't break. Once we got to the point in our journey where we needed to decrease plastic usage, I taught the kids one rule, never ever microwave anything in plastic. My biggest challenge was, you guessed it, the husband. He had to have the plastic microwave splatter cover with every microwave use. He could not be bothered to put leftovers on a plate. I can still remember one of the kids running across the kitchen, yelling, "Daddy, Daddy, stop microwaving in plastic! You will get cancer!" Drastic times called for drastic measures.

Let me begin by saying that plastic should be avoided. Period. If we are going to be honest, for most of us it's nearly impossible to cut it out completely. I have put together a chart to help you navigate this confusing world and to help you understand which type of plastic is safer and which types are really concerning.

You may have seen the following symbols on different containers. These signs were originally designed to identify which types of plastics could be recycled and reused. The chart below explains these numbers in depth. Of note, plastics can leach chemicals, particularly if exposed to sun, heat, repeated use, and abrasives.

Safer Plastics by the Numbers			
Avoid	Caution	Safest	
	1 PETE		Soft drinks, water bottles, nut butter jars - These are usually deemed safe but, because arsenic is used in manufacturing, proceed with caution. These are single-use so recycle them but do not re-use them.
		2 HDPE	Milk jugs, juice bottles, and detergent bottles - These are considered the safest, and most stable.
3 V			Cling film, food wrap, PVC pipe, teething rings, and toys - A major source of phthalates. These should be avoided.
		4 LDPE	Frozen food bags, squeezable bottles, and cling wrap - Consider replacing zipper food storage bags with silicone bags
		5 PP	Reusable microwaveable ware, kitchen ware, disposable plates, and cups - More heat resistant than others and therefor considered safer.
6 PS			Styrofoam cups, plates, and disposable takeout boxes - Avoid completely.
7 OTHER			Beverage bottles, baby bottles, electronic casings - Some may say BPA free. Call the company to find out what material is used and if it contains BP and BPF instead.

BPA

- BPA (Bisphenol A) is a chemical compound found in many things in our everyday lives. Some of them may even surprise you. The Mayo clinic has shown a direct correlation between children exposed to BPA and the development of ADHD. [1]

- Scientists at Mayo clinic have also found a correlation between BPA and myocarditis (an inflammatory condition of the heart generally caused by a virus) in rats. [2]

- High level maternal BPA exposure was shown to cause wheezing and affect the lung health of children born to pregnant women in Europe. [3]

Where is BPA found?

- BPA is found in plastic bottles, canned food, children's toys, hard food containers, and much more, and has been associated with adverse health effects, such as breast cancer, infertility, and childhood neurologic disorders. [4]

Items that Contain BPA	
Canned food	Fax paper
Canned Beverages	medical plastics and tubing
Canned liquid infant formula	Pacifier Shields
CDs	Plastic baby bottles
Cell phones	Plastic laboratory equipment
Children's toys	Plastic tableware
Coated paper used in receipts	Plastic water bottles
Dental sealants	Recycled paper products
DVD's	White dental fillings

Adapted from: https://www.clinicaladvisor.com/home/features/what-is-bpa-and-how-harmful-is-it-to-kids/

Fun BPA Facts

- In 2012, the FDA banned it from baby bottles and sippy cups.

- BPA-free does not mean it's safe. Replacement chemicals may be equally toxic. Animal studies show that replacements such as BPS, BPAF, BPZ have a significant impact on hormones and fertility. Unfortunately, companies in the US are still allowed to create chemicals without demonstrating safety. [5, 6]

Ways to reduce your BPA exposure

Four million tons of BPA are produced every year and there is widespread exposure to these compounds. No safe level of exposure has been established.

Cans

- Try not to buy foods in a can. If you must, make sure that the can has BPA-free lining and is not dented.

Receipts are covered in BPA

- At the grocery store, don't take the receipt. How often are you returning groceries?

- If you need it, have the receipt emailed to you.

Food Storage

- Containers and water bottles should be made of metal and glass.

- If this is not economically possible, using BPA-free products is not the perfect answer, but it's a start.

- Never microwave food in plastic containers of any kind. Heated plastic leaks toxic chemicals into food which goes directly into children's brains, potentially leading to ADHD.

Plastic is everywhere! Do the best you can.
1. Stop handling receipts.
2. Never ever microwave food
in anything plastic.

For my mega list of shopping items from Costco, Walmart, Trader Joe's, Target, Aldi, etc. scan the code for my book resources page.

31

I'll Take Mine Sunny Side Up

The Nitty-Gritty on Cookware

Where do I even begin with this story? Let's discuss the tantrum my husband threw when I tossed the non-stick pans. His award-winning dinner has always been bacon and eggs. My kids never fail to be thrilled when daddy cooks. If I am being honest, it's a bit annoying. I mean, I used to cook 99% of the meals which were often met with quiet pouting and hidden eyebrow raises. But when he managed to open a package of nitrite-free, humanely raised bacon and crack a couple of eggs into a toxic pan, the family rejoiced like it was Christmas. Thus, when the Teflon pan was put on the chopping block, John suspected revenge. Well, we have moved on from that conspiracy theory, but fear not, there is a lot of complaining about the cast iron pan which requires tender loving care to prevent scorched eggs.

Green, non-toxic cookware is as important as clean eating and organic food. It is one more thing to help us reduce our toxic load. What the heck does this mean? The body keeps count of all the processed food, poor sleep, uncontrolled stress, lack of movement, and environmental toxins. These things make up our toxic load. As we approach the end of the book, we cannot leave out cookware. Stay with me for 4 more pages.

MATERIALS THAT YOU SHOULD AVOID WHENEVER POSSIBLE:

- Teflon/non-stick
- Aluminum
- Plastic
- Clay
- Copper

Teflon

It is of the utmost importance to avoid nonstick cookware, also known as Teflon, which is generally made using poly- and perfluoroalkyl substances (PFAS). These substances release perfluorooctanoic acid (PFOA). Studies indicate that PFOA and PFOS can cause immune system issues and:

- Low sperm counts and small penises in humans [1]
- Developmental problems, liver and kidney issues, and immunological effects in laboratory animals [2]
- Tumors in animal studies [3]
- Low infant birth weights [4]
- Cancer [5]
- Thyroid hormone disruption [6]

Aluminum

The concern over aluminum pans is that it increases the total body burden of aluminum, leading to neurological issues like Alzheimer's disease, Parkinson's, and Multiple Sclerosis. [7] The data is mixed about aluminum toxicity in bakeware. I find it easier to err on the side of caution rather than later discover that I could have prevented neurological disease or cancer. To be safe, I made these changes:

- Instead of cooking on aluminum foil, I use non-bleached parchment paper.
- I do use aluminum foil to cover meats off the grill on big platters.
- I don't bake in the cheap disposable aluminum trays.

Plastic

This is addressed in the previous chapter.

Clay

Clay pots are made from, well, clay which is a natural product dug from the earth. It can contain heavy metals and toxins that have leached into water, soil, rock. When clay pots are created, various mixtures are used to form the ideal clay concoction. Traditional clay pots are not glazed so leaching of chemicals into food can occur:

- Arsenic was found to leach 10% more from unglazed pots. [8]
- Lead, cadmium, and iron can leach in considerable amounts from unglazed cookware. [9]
- Lead was used in glazes to make the product shinier and brighter. This is no longer the case, but if the pots are old or from China, beware.

Copper

The pots must be lined with stainless steel or tin to be safe. If the coating gets scratched, copper may leak into your food. Elevated copper levels have been seen with:

- Idiopathic copper toxicosis – diagnosed in infants and children across the world and caused by high concentrations of copper in drinking water or food. [10]
- Indian childhood cirrhosis – a liver disease found in infants in India who drank milk stored in copper pots. [10]

- Alzheimer's disease - elevations of copper in blood and the brain have been associated with the development of this disease. [10]
- An increased risk for postpartum depression. [11]

THE CAUTION MATERIALS:

- Cast iron
- Steel
- Glazed bakeware
- Silicone

Cast Iron

Seasoned cast iron pans are great. They can leach iron, which is okay for some foods. Don't simmer acidic foods like tomato sauce in this type of pan.

Steel

Stainless steel is also a good option, though there are some concerns with nickel and chromium leaching. This may be an issue for sensitive people [1]

Glazed

Again, glazed bakeware from China is at high risk of containing lead, as are old clay pots. If you are worried about lead in your product, you can obtain lead testing kits from online sources.

Silicone

Silicone appears to be safe. It is an inert material, meaning nothing used in its manufacturing will leach into foods. So far, no safety problems have been reported when used as molds. Stick to silicone kitchen tools, such as spatulas. Avoid silicone bakeware:

- Silicone bakeware when used at temperatures above 200° F has been shown to release volatile organic compounds (VOCs) and formaldehyde into your air and siloxanes into food. [12]

NON-TOXIC MATERIALS:

- Carbon steel
- Ceramic
- Lava rock
- Porcelain enamel
- Tempered glass

My 5 cookware items are:
- **Stainless steel: Instant Pot, saucepans and soup pot**
- **Ceramic: slow cooker, Caraway frying pan**
- **Glass bakeware**
- **Glazed iron: Le Creuset cast iron soup pot**
- **Cast iron frying pan**

For my mega list of shopping items from Costco, Walmart, Trader Joe's, Target, Aldi, etc. scan the code for my book resources page.

Acknowledgments

I can't believe I've finished writing my first book. This book has been in the making for 12 years. There are no words to describe how grateful I am for all the help I received along the way. But let me give it a go.

This book would have never happened without my husband John. If you would have told me 10 years ago that we would be writing a book together, I would have walked out of that room. But here we are Johnny T. I couldn't have done it without you. Somehow, I convinced you to be my editor, my publisher, book designer, and chart creator. While going through this journey, you rocked my world with Instant Pot creations, folded piles of laundry, a clean apartment, and taking care of the kids so I can focus on the task at hand. Truth be told, I love that orthopedic surgery has become your side gig. I am grateful every day for your love and support. You are my everything.

To my kids, Allie, Jake, and Evan: I love you all to the moon and back and I couldn't be prouder of the lovely young adults you are all becoming. You are all my greatest medical accomplishment.

To my parents, Cristina and Serban Marinescu: Thank you for making all the incredible sacrifices that come with emigration and settling into a new country. In this land of opportunity, a young girl got the chance to become a woman who will change the world for children everywhere. My only regret is that my father passed away before he could see me realize my dreams of becoming a doctor, with my own clinic, and my own book.

To my editor-in-chief, Jen: Thank you for the hours you spent reading and re-reading the never-ending added content. The organization of the citations alone requires a page of gratitude. Thanks for putting up with me and all of my continuous requests. I couldn't have done this project without you.

To my clinic team, Karen, Kelley, Anne, Brittney, and Lindsay: Thank you all for all the love and care you provide to our families. I learn something new from each and every one of you every single day. Without your help and support the clinic would not be standing, our online families would have been lost, and this book would have never been written. You are all a blessing to so many.

To all the families: There is no greater honor than a parent trusting me to care for their child. I applaud your commitment to keep your children healthy despite the odds. To all those who have struggled and are struggling to reverse their children's chronic disease, I admire your determination and perseverance, and I am grateful to be part of your journey.

To my social media tribe: @TheguthealthMD, Will Bulsiewicz, MD, thank you for writing such an incredible book, Fiber Fueled. Your book came out when I was feeling stuck in my writing. It not only provided me with incredible knowledge, but great inspiration. @foodbabe Vani Hari, for opening my eyes to ingredients in food and all the food industry's shenanigans. @plateful.health Vivian Chen, MD, for delivering amazing content that has influenced my posts, my research and this book. @chiefspicemama, Kanchan Koya, PhD for showing me that self-publishing can be done successfully and gracefully. You are the reason Indian spices are part of my cooking repertoire. And I can go on and on for pages. I have developed so many great friendships, connections, and have met so many wonderful people on a mission to change the world. Thank you to all my followers who not only support me but challenge me every day to dig deeper into the research, challenge the status quo, and be a louder voice for the children.

References

THE CURRENT STATE OF CHILDREN'S HEALTH

1. https://pubmed.ncbi.nlm.nih.gov/20159870/

2. https://www.cdc.gov/pcd/issues/2015/14_0397.htm

3. https://www.cdc.gov/pcd/issues/2015/14_0397.htm

4. Data and Statistics About ADHD. (2019, October 15). Retrieved from http//www.cdc.gov/ncbddd/adhd/data.html

5. Data & Statistics on Autism Spectrum Disorder. (2019, September 3). Retrieved from http//www.cdc.gov/ncbddd/autism/data.html

6. Childhood Obesity Facts (2019, June 24). Retrieved from http//cdc.gov/obesity/data/childhood.html

7. Data and Statistics on Children's Mental Health (2019, April 19). Retrieved from http//cdc.gov/childrensmentalhealth/data.html

8. Food Allergies (2019, May 29). Retrieved from http//www.cdc.gov/healthy-schools/foodallergies/index.html

9. Fast Stats-Asthma (2017, January 19). Retrieved from http//.cdc.gov/nchs/faststats/asthma.htm

10. https://pubmed.ncbi.nlm.nih.gov/20159870/

IMMUNE SYSTEM

1. https://www.britannica.com/science/neutrophil#:~:text=The%20bone%20marrow%20of%20a,after%20migrating%20to%20the%20tissues.

2. https://www.britannica.com/science/lymphocyte

3. https://www.sciencedirect.com/topics/immunology-and-microbiology/basophil-granulocyte#:~:text=Basophils%20differentiate%20from%20myeloid%20stem,et%20al.%2C%202011).

4. https://www.labce.com/spg538084_eosinophil_function_and_lifespan.aspx#:~:text=Eosinophils%20have%20a%20circulating%20half,so%20less%20readily%20than%20neutrophils.

PILLAR 1 NUTRITION

1. https://www.britannica.com/science/neutrophil#:~:text=The%20bone%20 marrow%20of%20a,after%20migrating%20to%20the%20tissues.

2. https://www.britannica.com/science/lymphocyte#:~:text=Most%20lympho-cytes%20are%20short%2Dlived,encounter%20with%20the%20same%20 antigen.

3. https://www.ncbi.nlm.nih.gov/pmc/articles/ PMC3903395/#:~:text=Unlike%20the%20lifespan%20of%20other,-days49%2C%2057%2C%2058.

4. https://www.ncbi.nlm.nih.gov/pmc/articles/ PMC5293177/#:~:text=Eosinophils%20are%20bone%20 marrow%E2%80%93derived,for%20at%20least%20several%20weeks.

5. https://www.ncbi.nlm.nih.gov/pmc/articles/PMC7352291/5a. https://gut. bmj.com/content/70/11/2096

6. https://academic.oup.com/ajcn/article-abstract/26/11/1180/4732762

7. https://pubmed.ncbi.nlm.nih.gov/18469238/

8. https://www.sciencedirect.com/science/article/abs/pii S0301054616301173

9. https://pubmed.ncbi.nlm.nih.gov/10728925/#

10. http://www.silcom.com/~dwsmith/midear.html

11. https://academic.oup.com/jn/article-abstract/125/5/1211/4730615?redirect-edFrom=fulltext

CHAPTER 1

1. https://onlinelibrary.wiley.com/doi/abs/10.1002/cd.155

2. https://onlinelibrary.wiley.com/doi/abs/10.1111/jpc.12428

3. https://jandonline.org/article/S0002-8223(07)01292-8/abstract

CHAPTER 2

1. https://www.canr.msu.edu/news/brain_nutrition_is_food_for_thought#:~:-text=The%20human%20brain%20uses%20about,how%20nutrition%20 affects%20the%20brain%3F

CHAPTER 3

1. http://uncfoodresearchprogram.web.unc.edu/poti-processed-foods-grocery/

CHAPTER 7

1. https://www.jpeds.com/article/S0022-3476(06)80164-2/abstract

CHAPTER 8

1. https://www.ncbi.nlm.nih.gov/pubmed/3312372

2. https://www.ncbi.nlm.nih.gov/pubmed/9215242

3. https://www.ncbi.nlm.nih.gov/pmc/articles/PMC2802046/

4. https://www.ewg.org/agmag/2015/06/big-corn-and-soy-go-defensive-cancer-experts-probe-dow-s-enlist-duo

5. https://www.fda.gov/food/food-additives-petitions/final-determination-regarding-partially-hydrogenated-oils-removing-trans-fat

6. http://www.themilkweed.com/Pizza_Cheese_Update_March_2006.pdf

7. https://www.sciencedirect.com/science/article/pii/S1382668918301571

CHAPTER 10

1. https://www.mayoclinic.org/healthy-lifestyle/nutrition-and-healthy-eating/in-depth/organic-food/art-20043880

2. https://www.mayoclinic.org/healthy-lifestyle/nutrition-and-healthy-eating/in-depth/organic-food/art-20043880

3. https://pubmed.ncbi.nlm.nih.gov/22430502/

4. https://www.ncbi.nlm.nih.gov/pmc/articles/PMC2846864/

5. https://health.clevelandclinic.org/when-going-organic-matters-most-for-you/

6. https://www.ncbi.nlm.nih.gov/pmc/articles/PMC3881124/

7. https://pubmed.ncbi.nlm.nih.gov/9113024/

8. https://www.intechopen.com/books/pesticides-in-the-modern-world-effects-of-pesticides-exposure/pesticide-exposure-of-farmworkers-children

9. https://www.ncbi.nlm.nih.gov/pmc/articles/PMC5813803/

10. https://www.tandfonline.com/doi/abs/10.1080/1354750X.2017.1395080

11. https://www.ncbi.nlm.nih.gov/pmc/articles/PMC3706632/

12. https://www.ncbi.nlm.nih.gov/pmc/articles/PMC4247335/

13. https://pubmed.ncbi.nlm.nih.gov/27992317/

14. https://www.sciencedirect.com/science/article/pii/S0160412012001341

15. https://ehjournal.biomedcentral.com/articles/10.1186/1476-069X-10-79

16. https://link.springer.com/article/10.1186/1476-069X-9-71

17. https://journals.lww.com/co-pediatrics/Abstract/2008/04000/Pesticides_and_child_neurodevelopment.16.aspx

18. https://www.sciencedirect.com/science/article/pii/S0013935119300246

19. https://www.ncbi.nlm.nih.gov/pmc/articles/PMC4947579/

20. https://pubmed.ncbi.nlm.nih.gov/25965039/

CHAPTER 12

1. https://www.who.int/news-room/q-a-detail/q-a-on-the-carcinogenicity-of-the-consumption-of-red-meat-and-processed-meat

2. https://foodanimalconcernstrust.org/food-labels/?gclid=EAIaIQobChMIvYzrm7CQ6gIVSuG1Ch1loAweEAAYBCAAEgKeMfD_BwE

3. https://www.consumerreports.org/cro/food/how-safe-is-your-ground-beef

4. https://www.mayoclinic.org/healthy-lifestyle/nutrition-and-healthy-eating/in-depth/organic-food/art-20043880

5. https://pubmed.ncbi.nlm.nih.gov/22430502/

6. https://www.ncbi.nlm.nih.gov/pmc/articles/PMC2846864/

7. https://health.clevelandclinic.org/when-going-organic-matters-most-for-you/

8. https://www.sciencedirect.com/science/article/pii/S1319562X17300049

9. https://www.ncbi.nlm.nih.gov/pmc/articles/PMC3194830/

10. https://www.ncbi.nlm.nih.gov/pmc/articles/PMC1804117/

11. https://pubmed.ncbi.nlm.nih.gov/14679840/

12. https://www.ncbi.nlm.nih.gov/pmc/articles/PMC4638249/

13. https://www.ncbi.nlm.nih.gov/books/NBK216502/

14. https://pubmed.ncbi.nlm.nih.gov/10366402/

15. https://www.webmd.com/food-recipes/news/20120106/antibiotics-food-animals-faq#1

16. https://www.mayoclinic.org/healthy-lifestyle/nutrition-and-healthy-eating/in-depth/organic-food/art-20043880

17. https://www.hsph.harvard.edu/news/press-releases/processed-meats-unprocessed-heart-disease-diabetes/#:~:text=Boston%2C%20MA%E2%80%94In%20a%20new,risk%20of%20type%202%20diabetes.

CHAPTER 14

1. https://olivecenter.ucdavis.edu/media/files/oliveoilfinal071410updated.pdf

2. https://www.sciencedirect.com/science/article/pii/S0956713520302449?via%3Dihub

3. https://www.futurity.org/avocado-oil-2388152/

CHAPTER 15

1. https://health.clevelandclinic.org/how-you-can-avoid-low-level-arsenic-in-rice-and-chicken/

2. https://pdfs.semanticscholar.org/fd43/051a2ef3682f323ce21cd0314e-a924e7b156.pdf

3. https://pubmed.ncbi.nlm.nih.gov/17384779/

4. https://www.consumerreports.org/cro/magazine/2015/01/how-much-arsenic-is-in-your-rice/index.htm

5. https://www.ncbi.nlm.nih.gov/pmc/articles/PMC1892142/#:~:text=A%20white%20rice%20sample%20from,soaks%20up%20arsenic%2C%20says%20Meharg.

6. https://www.consumerreports.org/cro/magazine/2015/01/how-much-arsenic-is-in-your-rice/index.htm

7. https://www.consumerreports.org/cro/magazine/2015/01/how-much-arsenic-is-in-your-rice/index.htm#rules

8. https://pubmed.ncbi.nlm.nih.gov/26515534/

9. https://pubmed.ncbi.nlm.nih.gov/19137137/

10. https://www.consumerreports.org/arsenic-in-food/arsenic-in-your-juice-apple-juice-grape-juice/

11. https://www.webmd.com/diet/news/20111130/arsenic-in-apple-grape-juice#1

12. https://www.webmd.com/diet/features/arsenic-food-faq#1

13. https://www.fda.gov/food/chemical-metals-natural-toxins-pesticides-guidance-documents-regulations/supporting-document-action-level-arsenic-apple-juice#:~:text=The%2010%20micrograms%2Fkilogram%20(%C2%B5g,and%20protective%20of%20public%20health.

CHAPTER 16

1. MedlinePlus

CHAPTER 17

1. https://pediatrics.aappublications.org/content/142/2/e20181408

2. http://sitn.hms.harvard.edu/flash/2015/the-flavor-rundown-natural-vs-artificial-flavors/

3. https://www.ewg.org/research/ewg-s-dirty-dozen-guide-food-additives/food-colors-questions-and-contamination

4. https://hub.jhu.edu/2015/02/19/soda-caramel-coloring-cancer/

5. https://www.ewg.org/research/ewg-s-dirty-dozen-guide-food-additives/food-additives-linked-health-risks#potassiumbromate

6. https://www.ewg.org/research/ewg-s-dirty-dozen-guide-food-additives/food-additives-linked-health-risks#potassiumbromate

7. https://www.ewg.org/research/ewg-s-dirty-dozen-guide-food-additives/generally-recognized-as-safe-but-is-it#butylated-hydroxyanisole

8. https://www.ewg.org/research/ewg-s-dirty-dozen-guide-food-additives/generally-recognized-as-safe-but-is-it#butylated-hydroxyanisole

9. https://www.ewg.org/research/ewg-s-dirty-dozen-guide-food-additives/generally-recognized-as-safe-but-is-it#butylated-hydroxyanisole

10. https://msutoday.msu.edu/news/2016/common-additive-may-be-why-you-have-food-allergies/

11. https://pubchem.ncbi.nlm.nih.gov/compound/Propyl-gallate#:~:text=Propyl%20gallate%20is%20found%20in,Especially%20effective%20with%20polyunsaturated%20fats.

12. https://www.ewg.org/research/ewg-s-dirty-dozen-guide-food-additives/generally-recognized-as-safe-but-is-it#butylated-hydroxyanisole

13. https://www.ewg.org/research/ewg-s-dirty-dozen-guide-food-additives/fda-failed-us

CHAPTER 18

1. https://www.frontiersin.org/articles/10.3389/fped.2020.00058/full

2. https://kids.frontiersin.org/articles/10.3389/frym.2019.00032

3. https://pubmed.ncbi.nlm.nih.gov/28274718/

4. https://www.ncbi.nlm.nih.gov/pmc/articles/PMC7230400/

5. https://www.ncbi.nlm.nih.gov/pmc/articles/PMC4563885/

6. https://www.ncbi.nlm.nih.gov/pmc/articles/PMC4876724/

7. https://www.sciencedaily.com/releases/2021/03/210331130910.htm

8. https://www.sciencedirect.com/science/article/abs/pii/S0306452202001239?via%3Dihub

9. https://pubmed.ncbi.nlm.nih.gov/32356872/

10. https://pubmed.ncbi.nlm.nih.gov/31311146/

11. https://www.ncbi.nlm.nih.gov/pmc/articles/PMC7312722/

12. https://www.ncbi.nlm.nih.gov/pmc/articles/PMC6627124/

13. https://www.mdpi.com/1420-3049/25/22/5480

14. https://www.ncbi.nlm.nih.gov/pmc/articles/PMC7008860/

PILLAR II STRESS

1. https://www.ncbi.nlm.nih.gov/pmc/articles/PMC1361287/

2. https://pubmed.ncbi.nlm.nih.gov/8610165/

3. https://www.scientificamerican.com/article/stress-can-weaken-vaccine/

4. https://pubmed.ncbi.nlm.nih.gov/9619470/

5. https://d1wqtxts1xzle7.cloudfront.net/70684/1ah1j1rcta-4ajx95st99.pdf?1425067516=&response-content-disposition=inline%3B+filename%3DLink_to_full_text_pdf.pdf&Expires=1598355262&Signature=DCSTE-H-oIapvmjHbbIsDe-mOw-dvC9WCIo0YAtaD4behW-rXGuSD5p55MMyFRY9-n761p0GzT-tOp20h-ZehazqM-crT0jFo9LPPszhZPSTTWtUB0UYk06FyBzVT18e5rG-DQLhtzFDSNXIZ6Tu7PPIYjFGiChlcwoVpxrjDTxldB7xpCBawpo4Bt3G thIXOfNyiXU3oSaJyl0jUDmfeLvZtMEvGxmLywABflMCYWUDvzvL0oo Bp-37z-vLhZyyQvzATBwf2FlTtTbbZTZHaEdo95yA3RNMTNvHdbgG -YjN2r--tLBVlMO21-2pOHm6mcOvQ0XnTbExFx87I1-XX0gSA__& Key-Pair-Id=APKAJLOHF5GGSLRBV4ZA

6. https://www.ncbi.nlm.nih.gov/pmc/articles/PMC4225959/

7. https://pubmed.ncbi.nlm.nih.gov/9200634/

8. https://www.discovermagazine.com/health/can-stress-loneliness-and-sleep-deprivation-make-you-more-prone-to-covid-19

CHAPTER 23

1. https://jamanetwork.com/journals/jamainternalmedicine/fullarticle/1809754

2. https://www.ncbi.nlm.nih.gov/pmc/articles/PMC3092730/

3. https://pubmed.ncbi.nlm.nih.gov/21105176/

4. https://www.ncbi.nlm.nih.gov/pmc/articles/PMC4280720/

5. https://www.ncbi.nlm.nih.gov/pmc/articles/PMC4270653/

6. https://pubmed.ncbi.nlm.nih.gov/25553641/

7. https://pubmed.ncbi.nlm.nih.gov/17211115/

8. https://pubmed.ncbi.nlm.nih.gov/22894890/

9. https://pubmed.ncbi.nlm.nih.gov/18753801/

10. https://pubmed.ncbi.nlm.nih.gov/22849536/

11. https://pubmed.ncbi.nlm.nih.gov/33463729/

PILLAR III SLEEP

1. https://www.ncbi.nlm.nih.gov/pmc/articles/PMC2629403/

2. https://www.ncbi.nlm.nih.gov/pmc/articles/PMC3242694/

3. https://www.researchgate.net/publication/11146743_Effect_of_sleep_deprivation_on_response_to_immunizaton

4. https://www.sciencedaily.com/releases/2019/02/190212094839.htm

CHAPTER 24

1. https://www.ncbi.nlm.nih.gov/pmc/articles/PMC7324339/

2. https://onlinelibrary.wiley.com/doi/10.1002/rmv.2109

3. https://www.ncbi.nlm.nih.gov/pmc/articles/PMC5454613/

4. https://www.health.harvard.edu/blog/cell-phone-use-stimulates-brain-activity-201102231548

5. https://jamanetwork.com/journals/jama/fullarticle/645813

6. Murphy PJ, Campbell SS. Nighttime drop in body temperature: a physiological trigger for sleep onset? Sleep. 1997 Jul; 20(7): 505-11.

PILLAR IV MOVEMENT

1. https://www.ncbi.nlm.nih.gov/pmc/articles/
   PMC2092583/#:~:text=Strenuous%20physical%20activity%20at%20
   least,and%20intensity%20of%20physical%20activity.

2. https://bjsm.bmj.com/content/45/12/987.abstract?sid=e6594508-3aaa-
   4c61-99ba-4ea138580947

3. https://www.researchgate.net/profile/David_Nieman/publica-
   tion/20868569_The_Effects_of_Moderate_Exercise_Training_on_
   Natural_Killer_Cells_and_Acute_Upper_Respiratory_Tract_Infections/
   links/55670c0d08aeab77721e639f.pdf

4. https://journals.sagepub.com/doi/10.2466/pr0.94.3.839-844

5. McCarthy DA, Macdonald I, Grant M et al. Studies on the immediate and
   delayed leucocytosis elicited by brief (30-min) strenuous exercise. Eur J Appl
   Physiol1992;64:513–7.

6. http://www.bio.umass.edu/micro/immunology/540sigs/exercise.htm

7. https://pubmed.ncbi.nlm.nih.gov/18461130/

8. https://medlineplus.gov/ency/article/007165.htm

9. https://www.thieme-connect.com/products/ejournals/abstract/
   10.1055/s-2007-1021134

Chapter 25

1. http://www.pollyklaas.org/about/national-child-kidnapping.html

2. https://www.savethechildren.org/us/charity-stories/child-trafficking-myths-
   vs-facts

3. https://www.americanbar.org/groups/public_interest/child_law/resources/
   child_law_practiceonline/child_law_practice/vol-34/november-2015/risk-
   factors-for-child-trafficking/

PILLAR V ENVIRONMENT

1. https://cen.acs.org/articles/95/i9/chemicals-use-today.html#:~:text=No%20
   one%2C%20not%20even%20the,Substances%20Control%20Act%20
   (TSCA).

2. http://www.safecosmetics.org/get-the-facts/regulations/internation-
   al-laws/#:~:text=The%20EU%20law%20bans%201%2C328,restricted%20
   11%20chemicals%20from%20cosmetics.

3. https://pubmed.ncbi.nlm.nih.gov/25838260/

4. https://pubmed.ncbi.nlm.nih.gov/29451393/

5. https://www.ncbi.nlm.nih.gov/pmc/articles/
PMC3060004/#:~:text=Okada%20et%20al.-,2010).,2010).

6. https://www.ewg.org/news/news-releases/2008/05/13/major-study-teflon-chemical-people-suggests-harm-immune-system-liver

7. https://jamanetwork.com/journals/jama/fullarticle/1104903

8. https://ehp.niehs.nih.gov/doi/10.1289/ehp.1307670

CHAPTER 26

1. Janjua 2004, Janjua 2008, Sarveiya 2004, Gonzalez 2006, Rodriguez 2006, Krause 2012, Ghazipura 2017, Matta 2020.

2. Krause 2012, Sarveiya 2004, Rodriguez 2006, Klinubol 2008, Matta 2020.

3. "https://www.ncbi.nlm.nih.gov/pmc/articles/PMC6312469/"3 Krause 2012, Sarveiya 2004, SCCNFP 2006, Matta 2020.

4. Walters 1997, Shaw 2006, Singh 2007, Matta 2020.

5. Krause 2012, Bryden 2006, Hayden 2005, Matta 2020.

6. Klinubol 2008, Bryden 2006, Hayden 2005, Montenegro 2008, Nash 2014, Matta 2020.

7. Berger KP, et al. HERMOSA study. J Expo Sci Environ Epidemiol 29(1):21-32.

8. Smith KW, et al . Environ Health Perspect 121(11-12):1299-305.

9. **Nishihama Y**, et al 2016. **Reprod Toxicol** 63:107-13

10. **Geer LA, et al.** J Hazard Mater 323(Pt A):177-183.

11. Gynecol **Endocrinol.** 2019, Reprod Toxicol. (2016), Dr Swan 1999

12. https://ec.europa.eu/health/scientific_committees/consumer_safety/docs/sccs_o_199.pdf

ADDITIONAL SUNSCREEN RESOURCES

1. https://www.ewg.org/sunscreen/report/the-trouble-with-sunscreen-chemicals/

2. https://www.ncbi.nlm.nih.gov/pmc/articles/PMC6312469/

3. https://www.ewg.org/californiacosmetics/parabens

4. National Toxicology Program 2012

CHAPTER 27

1. https://pubmed.ncbi.nlm.nih.gov/12900480/

2. https://www.ncbi.nlm.nih.gov/pmc/articles/PMC4125160/

3. https://www.atsdr.cdc.gov/phs/phs.asp?id=1447&tid=201

4. https://www.atsdr.cdc.gov/toxprofiles/tp.asp?id=1451&tid=201

5. https://www.canada.ca/en/health-canada/services/about-pesticides/insect-repellents.html

6. https://academic.oup.com/jtm/article/25/suppl_1/S10/4990399
   https://www3.epa.gov/pesticides/chem_search/reg_actions/registration/fs_PC-070705_01-May-05.pdf

7. https://www.ewg.org/research/ewgs-guide-bug-repellents/repellent-chemicals?_ga=2.94598684.1055855279.1600031563-227777591.1588451792&_gac=1.127318271.1600032270.Cj0KCQjwhvf6BRCkARIsAGl1GGhxeUjvRiAg1Yb1pf_FImNagzEnbHLr5Kmt6A2-Qsw04zgx6e69yEoaAtXJEALw_wcB&_gl=1*s16tzj*_gcl_aw*R0NMLjE2MDAwMzIyNzAuQ2owS0NRandodmY2QlJDa0FSSXNBR2wxR0doeGVVanZSaUFnMVliMXBmX0ZJbmJJITHI1S210NkEyLVFzdzA0emd4NmU2OXlFb2FBdFhKRUFMd193Y0I.#4

8. Registration of the Formulated Product Repel Lemon Eucalyptus (EPA Reg. No. 305-56) and the Manufacturing Use Product (MUP) (Reg. No. 305-59) Containing the New Active Ingredient Citriodiol. New York State Department of Environmental Conservation. May 16, 200

9. https://pubmed.ncbi.nlm.nih.gov/19815887/

CHAPTER 28

1. https://data.europa.eu/euodp/en/data/dataset/cosmetic-ingredient-database-2-list-of-substances-prohibited-in-cosmetic-products

CHAPTER 29

1. https://www.cdc.gov/mmwr/preview/mmwrhtml/rr5014a1.htm

2. https://dash.harvard.edu/bitstream/handle/1/10579664/3491930.

pdf?amp%3BisAllowed=y&sequence=1

3. https://www.cochranelibrary.com/cdsr/doi/10.1002/14651858.CD010856. pub2/full

4. https://pubmed.ncbi.nlm.nih.gov/31424532/

5. https://apps.who.int/iris/bitstream/handle/10665/112662/97892415487 00_eng.pdf

6. https://www.livestrong.com/article/532986-foods-containing-fluoride/

7. https://www.colgate.com/en-us/oral-health/basics/selecting-dental-products/ what-is-hydroxyapatite-toothpaste

8. https://www.ncbi.nlm.nih.gov/pmc/articles/PMC5390120/?_ ga=2.209293334.569157030.1600628762-1175999940.1600628762

9. https://www.researchgate.net/publication/275420895_Addition_ of_Hydroxyapatite_to_Toothpaste_and_Its_Effect_to_Dentin_ Remineralization

10. https://www.ncbi.nlm.nih.gov/pmc/articles/PMC5997847/?_ ga=2.55679663.569157030.1600628762-1175999940.1600628762

11. https://www.researchgate.net/profile/Subrata_Nath3/publica- tion/275420895_Addition_of_Hydroxyapatite_to_Toothpaste_and_Its_ Effect_to_Dentin_Remineralization/links/553c84760cf245bdd7668c1a.pdf

12. https://www.researchgate.net/profile/Bennett_Amaechi/publica- tion/221690050_Remineralization_of_early_caries_by_a_nano-hydroxyapa- tite_dentifrice/links/0fcfd502d03a6c7db7000000.pdf

13. https://www.ncbi.nlm.nih.gov/pmc/articles/PMC6901576/

14. https://pubmed.ncbi.nlm.nih.gov/15348313/

15. https://www.ncbi.nlm.nih.gov/pmc/articles/PMC4965058/

CHAPTER 30

1. https://www.sciencedirect.com/science/article/abs/pii/S0013935116302110

2. https://www.frontiersin.org/articles/10.3389/fendo.2019.00598/full

3. https://www.sciencedaily.com/releases/2019/10/191001094205.htm

4. https://pubmed.ncbi.nlm.nih.gov/25813067/#:~:text=Therefore%2C%20 BPA%20has%20been%20shown,polycystic%20ovary%20syndrome%20 (PCOS).

5.   https://www.sciencedaily.com/releases/2020/02/200218182202.htm

6.   https://www.nationalgeographic.com/science/2018/09/news-BPA-free-plastic-safety-chemicals-health/

CHAPTER 31

1.   https://assets.documentcloud.org/documents/5316830/EDCs-Androgenic-Activity-Perfluoroakyl.pdf

2.   https://www.ncbi.nlm.nih.gov/pmc/articles/PMC2679623/

3.   https://www.epa.gov/pfas/basic-information-pfas#:~:text=The%20most%2Dstudied%20PFAS%20chemicals,have%20caused%20tumors%20in%20animals.

4.   https://www.ncbi.nlm.nih.gov/pmc/articles/PMC2072861/

5.   https://www.cancer.org/cancer/cancer-causes/teflon-and-perfluorooctanoic-acid-pfoa.html

6.   https://www.ncbi.nlm.nih.gov/pmc/articles/PMC2866686/#:~:text=cause%20for%20concern.-,Conclusions,adult%20population%20representative%20study%20samples.

7.   https://www.frontiersin.org/articles/10.3389/fneur.2014.00212/full#:~:text=In%20the%20brain%2C%20aluminum%20will,of%20the%20brain%20(32).

8.   https://www.sciencedirect.com/science/article/abs/pii/S0048969711003846

9.   file:///Users/anatemple/Downloads/78893-Article%20Text-184476-1-10-20120712.pdf

10. https://www.ncbi.nlm.nih.gov/pmc/articles/PMC4113679/

11. https://pubmed.ncbi.nlm.nih.gov/17317521/

12. https://medium.com/@marycaldarelli/is-silicone-cookware-safe-bb812a4054f1

Printed in Poland
by Amazon Fulfillment
Poland Sp. z o.o., Wrocław

33687832R00148